Map Key

(Continued on next page)

Rocky
Mountain
National Park

Other Books by Kim Lipker

The Best in Tent Camping: Colorado (with Johnny Molloy)

60 Hikes within 60 Miles: Denver and Boulder

The Unofficial Guide to Bed & Breakfasts and Country Inns in the Rockies

DAY &OVERNIGHT HIKES

Rocky Mountain National Park

Kim Lipker

Menasha Ridge Press

DISCLAIMER

This book is meant only as a guide to select trails in the vicinity of the Rocky Mountain National Park and does not guarantee hiker safety in any way—you hike at your own risk. Neither Menasha Ridge Press nor Kim Lipker is liable for property loss or damage, personal injury, or death that result in any way from accessing or hiking the trails described in the following pages. Please be aware that hikers have been injured in the Rocky Mountain National Park area. Be especially cautious when walking on or near boulders, steep inclines, and drop-offs, and do not attempt to explore terrain that may be beyond your abilities. To help ensure an uneventful hike, please read carefully the introduction to this book, and perhaps get further safety information and guidance from other sources. Familiarize yourself thoroughly with the areas you intend to visit before venturing out. Ask questions, and prepare for the unforeseen. Familiarize yourself with current weather reports, maps of the area you intend to visit, and any relevant park regulations.

Published by Menasha Ridge Press
Printed in the United States of America
Distributed by Publishers Group West
First edition, first printing

♻ Printed on recycled paper

Text and cover design by Ian Szymkowiak/Palace Press International
Cover photograph © Daniel H. Bailey/Alamy
Photograph on page 25 © Kim Lipker
Photograph on page 145 © Bruce Becker
Cartography and elevation profiles by Kim Lipker and Scott McGrew
Indexing by Jan Mucciarone

Library of Congress Cataloging-in-Publication Data

Lipker, Kim, 1969–
    Day & overnight hikes, Rocky Mountain National Park/Kim Lipker. —1st ed.
      p. cm.
    Includes index.
    ISBN-13: 978-0-89732-655-1
    ISBN-10: 0-89732-655-5
    1. Hiking—Colorado—Rocky Mountain National Park—Guidebooks. 2. Rocky Mountain
National Park (Colo.)—Guidebooks. I. Title. II. Title: Day and overnight hikes, Rocky Mountain
National Park.
    GV199.42.C2L57 2008
    796.510978869—dc22

                        2008015760

Menasha Ridge Press
P.O. Box 43673
Birmingham, Alabama 35243
www.menasharidge.com

Table of Contents

EAST SIDE OF ROCKY MOUNTAIN NATIONAL PARK

NORTHEAST SIDE OF ROCKY MOUNTAIN NATIONAL PARK (NORTH FORK AREA AND MUMMY RANGE)

EAST CENTER OF ROCKY MOUNTAIN
NATIONAL PARK (GORGE LAKES AREA
AND BEAR LAKE AREA)

SOUTHEAST SIDE OF ROCKY MOUNTAIN
NATIONAL PARK (LONGS PEAK AREA
AND WILD BASIN AREA)

WEST SIDE OF ROCKY MOUNTAIN NATIONAL PARK

NORTHWEST SIDE OF ROCKY MOUNTAIN NATIONAL PARK (TRAIL RIDGE ROAD, COLORADO RIVER HEADWATERS AREA, AND NEVER SUMMER RANGE)

SOUTHWEST SIDE OF ROCKY MOUNTAIN NATIONAL PARK (TONAHUTU AREA, EAST INLET AREA, AND NORTH INLET AREA)

Dedication

For Karen Lipker, my favorite little sister. We'll always have good memories of Estes Park and the infamous "What does 'No Vacancy' mean?" family trip.

Acknowledgments

I cannot thank the following people enough! So . . . thank you
times infinity.

Abby Balfany
Bruce Becker
Michael Bollinger
Christa Gorman
Russell Helms
Nancy Stilson-Herzog
Lindsay Hopper
Jen Janssen
Kelly Josephs
Anna, Alex, and Emma Lipker
Ruth and Roger Lipker (Mom and Dad)
Molly Merkle
Johnny Molloy
Robert Muchow (Grandpa)
MaryAnn Muchow
Paul Muchow
Tricia Parks
Anne Perkins
Lindsay Smith and Paul Chavez
Diane Stanko and Marty Martinez
Murielle Watzky-Brewer
John and Fiona Wilson

Preface

Rocky Mountain National Park

The crowning jewel of anyone's hiking or backpacking history is Rocky Mountain National Park. That's why it is such an honor for me to write a book about an extraordinary national park that is right in my backyard. If you are lucky enough to live within driving distance of Rocky Mountain National Park, you know what I mean, and you'll also find the 30 hikes featured here may keep you busy for years to come.

Visitors to Colorado will most likely join thousands of others who make their way to Rocky Mountain National Park every year (3 million, to be exact). It is truly an experience not to be missed. More than 110 mountain peaks tower over the 415 square miles of hiking trails, picnic spots, waterfalls, cold lakes, and bountiful wildlife.

It was my job to narrow the aforementioned hiking trails and 269 backcountry campsites into useful recommendations for day hikes and overnight hikes in Rocky Mountain National Park. The selections were made based on a variety of criteria and are what make up this manageable and well-rounded guidebook.

Rocky Mountain National Park is located northwest of Denver, spanning Grand and Larimer counties and bordered on the west by the town of Grand Lake and on the east by the town of Estes Park. The park is revered by residents on Colorado's Western Slope and the Front Range. This is especially true of all of those that can see the towering peaks from their car windows when they drive around the northern part of the Colorado Front Range (Fort Collins to Boulder to Denver).

Adjacent to Indian Peaks Wilderness and Comanche Peaks Wilderness to the north and to Never Summer Wilderness to the west, the park is also surrounded by Routt, Roosevelt, and Arapaho national forests. Now is an exciting time for Rocky Mountain National Park because it's progressing toward wilderness designation. Rocky Mountain National Park has been a candidate for wilderness designation since the Wilderness Act was passed in 1964. The park was established by Congress in 1915 with the help of naturalist Enos Mills and F. O. Stanley. In 1974 President Nixon recommended 239,835 acres for wilderness designation, providing permanent protection for the park. The area has been managed as wilderness since the 1960s, its wilderness qualities protected and celebrated by several generations of park employees and park visitors.

The elevations in Rocky Mountain National Park range from 7,500 feet to 14,255 feet, encompassing green valleys and alpine tundra. Longs Peak is the highest peak, and Mount Meeker, at 13,911 feet, rises to the south. Seventy-two mountains exceed 12,000 feet, and more than 110 of the peaks soar above 10,000 feet. (That's almost 2 miles above sea level!) The valleys below these high peaks are thick with lodgepole-pine, juniper, and spruce forests and are rich with wildlife.

Rocky Mountain National Park is home to 150 lakes and plenty of rivers, streams, and waterfalls. The Colorado River marks its birthplace in the park. The Continental Divide runs northwest to southeast through the park. Snowmelt and rainwater to the west of the Great Divide flows toward the Pacific Ocean; runoff to the east is bound for the Gulf of Mexico and the Atlantic Ocean.

People are also a part of the Rocky Mountain National Park wilderness. Hikers, anglers, miners, homesteaders, pioneers, Native Americans, and more have made their way through the park's history.

During the research for this book, I became nostalgic for all the years I have spent in the park. My grandma, grandpa, aunt, cousin, and another aunt and uncle all live or have lived here. I've even lived in Estes Park. My cousin was married at the historic Stanley Hotel during the writing of this book. My grandpa also passed away during my last days of research, ten years to the month after my grandma died.

It was a joy to hike with my sister and recall the fun we've had in the park. This includes everything from her falling in the ashes of an old campfire (in the olden days of course) to hearing about Grandma's high-school senior trip to Longs Peak (in the way-olden days, the 1930s to be exact). In a way, the mountains are tied to Grandma, and not a day goes by that I don't think of her.

My respect for the management of the park has never waned. The trails here are constantly upgraded as are the facilities in and outside the park. You can be assured that even the pit toilets will be clean and always smelling fresh. I recommend visiting the area in the fall, when the elk are in the valleys for their bugling, or mating, season. Crowds are thinning, the colors are changing, and the weather is still quite pleasant.

Lesser-known hikes, such as the hikes on the west side of the park, were nice to revisit. These hikes tend to be longer and less crowded and are great for travelers spending a night or two around the Grand Lake area. Onahu Creek Trailhead: Onahu Creek Trail and Green Mountain Trail Loop is a perfect example. The other hikes in the southwest side of Rocky Mountain National Park are located in the Tonahutu, East Inlet, and North Inlet areas. These are hikes that border Grand Lake and travel through the other side of the park.

The best way to explore the history of Rocky Mountain National Park and the surrounding area is to visualize those people who have walked the trails before you. Pioneers who just crossed over the Continental Divide and claimed their homestead can be revisited on trails such as the Holzwarth Historic Site: Never Summer Ranch. Other hikes on the northwest side of Rocky Mountain National Park encompass the areas around Trail Ridge Road, Colorado River Headwaters, and the Never Summer Range. These trails range from flat meadow hikes to alpine tundra treks.

On the east side, you'll find some nice surprises among the old tried-and-true. An overall favorite hike of mine is Cow Creek Trailhead: Bridal Veil Falls. Other hikes on the northeast side of Rocky Mountain National Park are in the North Fork Area and the Mummy Range. These are four real winners! However, a couple did get lost on the trail to the Cache Campsite while I was writing this book. Be sure to take the book along if you go.

The East Center of Rocky Mountain National Park is the most crowded area of all: Gorge Lakes and Bear Lake. Creative timing, e.g., weekdays in the spring, fall, or winter, will make hikes like Bear Lake Trailhead: The Loch, well, bearable. All of the hikes in this region are unique in terrain and difficulty, thus their popularity.

On the southeast side of Rocky Mountain National Park is where you'll the find the infamous Longs Peak, along with the Wild Basin area. Be sure to try out lesser-known hikes here, such as Sandbeach Lake, which is another personal favorite.

If you're touring Estes Park, be sure to stop at the Stanley Hotel. My aunt has waitressed there for more than 20 years, and the hotel is rich with stories; they say that Stephen King found the inspiration for *The Shining* while staying here.

In the time that it took me to research and write this book, many people were lost and found while hiking in Rocky Mountain National Park. That serves as a reminder to please be careful on the trail and always hike with a buddy. At the very least, let someone know where you're going and when you expect to be back.

Thank you for buying or borrowing this book. Be assured that I had you, the reader, in mind during every one of my hikes. By picking up this book, you have also, by default become a steward of the wilderness and must make a pledge to preserve our national parks. I for one want my kids and generations that follow to experience the joy of Rocky Mountain National Park.

Recommended Hikes

DAY & OVERNIGHT HIKES

RECOMMENDED HIKES

DAY & OVERNIGHT HIKES

RECOMMENDED HIKES

DAY & OVERNIGHT HIKES

RECOMMENDED HIKES

Introduction

How to Use This Guidebook

The Overview Map and Overview-map Key

Use the overview map on the inside front cover to assess the exact locations of each hike's primary trailhead. Each hike's number appears on the overview map, on the map key facing the overview map, in the table of contents, and at the top of each trail map.

The book is organized by region, as indicated in the table of contents. The hikes within each region are noted as day hikes or overnight hikes in the map key and in the table of contents.

Trail Maps

Each hike contains a detailed map that shows the trailhead, the route, significant features, facilities, and topographic landmarks such as creeks, overlooks, and peaks. The author gathered map data by carrying a global-positioning-system (GPS) unit while hiking. This data was downloaded into a digital mapping program (DeLorme's Topo USA) and processed by expert cartographers to produce the highly accurate maps found in this book. Each trailhead's GPS coordinates are included with each profile (see next page).

Elevation Profiles

Corresponding to the trail map, each hike contains a detailed elevation profile that provides a quick look at the trail from the side, enabling you to visualize how the trail rises and falls. Key points along the way are labeled. Note the number of feet between each tick mark on the vertical axis (the height scale). To avoid making flat hikes look steep and steep hikes appear flat, height scales are used throughout the book to provide an accurate image of the hike's difficulty.

GPS TRAILHEAD COORDINATES

To collect accurate map data, each trail was hiked with a handheld GPS unit (Garmin eTrex). Data collected was then downloaded and plotted onto a digital U.S. Geological Survey topographic map. In addition to rendering highly specific trail outlines, this book also includes the GPS coordinates for each trailhead in Universal Transverse Mercator (UTM) format.

UTM coordinates index a specific point using a grid method (topo maps show UTM grid lines as well as latitude and longitude). The survey datum used to arrive at the coordinates in this book is WGS84. For readers who own a GPS unit, whether handheld or onboard a vehicle, the UTM coordinates provided on the first page of each hike may be entered into the unit. Just make sure that your GPS unit is set to navigate using WGS84 datum. Now you can navigate directly to the trailhead.

Most trailheads, which begin in parking areas, can be reached by car, but some hikes still require a short walk to reach the trailhead from a parking area. In those cases a handheld unit is necessary to continue the GPS navigation process. That said, however, readers can easily access all trailheads in this book by using the directions given, the overview map, and the trail map, which shows at least one major road leading into the area. But for those who enjoy using the latest GPS technology to navigate, the necessary data has been provided. A brief explanation of the UTM coordinates from Lawn Lake Trailhead: Ypsilon Trail to Upper Chipmunk Campsite (page 38) follows.

UTM Zone	13T
Easting	0446930
Northing	4472930

The UTM zone number 13 refers to one of the 60 vertical zones of the UTM projection. Each zone is 6 degrees wide. The UTM zone letter T refers to one of the 20 horizontal zones that span from 80 degrees south to 84 degrees north. The easting number **0446930** indicates in meters how far east or west a point is from the central meridian of the zone. Increasing easting coordinates on a topo map or on your GPS screen indicate that you are moving east; decreasing easting coordinates indicate you are moving west. The northing number **4472930** references in meters how far you are from the equator. Above and below the equator, increasing northing coordinates indicate you are traveling north, while decreasing northing coordinates indicate you are traveling south.

To learn more about how to enhance your outdoor experiences with GPS technology, refer to *GPS Outdoors: A Practical Guide for Outdoor Enthusiasts,* by Russell Helms (Menasha Ridge Press).

The Hike Profile

In addition to maps, each hike contains a concise but informative narrative of the hike from beginning to end. This descriptive text is enhanced with at-a-glance ratings and information, GPS-based trailhead coordinates, and accurate driving directions that lead you from a major road to the parking area that is most convenient to the trailhead.

At the top of the section for each hike is a box that allows the hiker quick access to pertinent information: quality of scenery, condition of trail, appropriateness for children, difficulty of hike, quality of solitude expected, hike distance, approximate hiking time, and outstanding highlights of the trip. The first five categories are rated using a five-star system. An example follows:

1 Cow Creek Trailhead: *Bridal Veil Falls*

Scenery: ☆ ☆ ☆ ☆	Distance: *6.44 mi. out-and-back*
Trail condition: ☆ ☆ ☆ ☆	Hiking time: *3.5 hours*
Children: ☆ ☆ ☆	Outstanding features: *Thundering waterfall; meadow and alpine landscape; historical ranch*
Difficulty: ☆ ☆ ☆	
Solitude: ☆ ☆ ☆	

The four stars in the first rating indicate that the scenery is picturesque. The trail condition, as shown in the next rating, is also four stars, or very good (one star would mean the trail is likely to be muddy, rocky, overgrown, or otherwise compromised). The hike is doable for able-bodied children, hence three stars (a one-star rating would denote that only the most gung-ho and physically fit kids should go).The three stars for difficulty denote that the hike is moderately challenging (five stars would mean much greater difficulty). The final rating of three stars means you can expect to encounter relatively few people on the trail (whereas with one star, you may well be elbowing your way along).

Distances given are absolute, but hiking times are estimated for an average hiking speed of 2 to 3 miles per hour, with time built in for pauses at overlooks and brief rests. Overnight-hiking times account for the effort of carrying a backpack.

Following each box is a brief italicized description of the hike. A more detailed account follows in which trail junctions, stream crossings, and trailside features are noted along with their distance from the trailhead. Flip through the book, read the descriptions, and choose a hike that appeals to you.

Weather

Rocky Mountain National Park weather is always changing. Temperatures drop, and precipitation increases proportionate to the altitude. The higher the elevation, the lower the temperature. Be prepared and dress in layers. Always prepare for chilly conditions. It's easier to take off a layer that you have than it is to add a layer that you don't have. At right is a quick snapshot of the weather in the area.

Temperature and Precipitation
(Temperatures are averages in degrees Fahrenheit.)

Estes Park (elevation 7,522')

	High	Low	Precipitation	Snow
Jan.	39	16	0.37"	4.6"
Feb.	41	17	0.45"	6.3"
March	45	21	0.86"	7.8"
April	53	27	1.28"	3.8"
May	62	34	2.02"	0.5"
June	73	41	1.76"	0.1"
July	78	46	2.21"	0.0"
Aug.	77	45	1.86"	0.0"
Sept.	70	38	1.17"	0.5"
Oct.	60	30	0.81"	1.0"
Nov.	46	23	0.60"	3.8"
Dec.	40	18	0.47"	5.7"

Grand Lake (elevation 8,369')

	High	Low	Precipitation	Snow
Jan.	31	2	1.68"	29.6"
Feb.	35	4	1.43"	22.5"
March	40	10	1.54"	19.5"
April	49	19	1.88"	16.8"
May	59	27	1.94"	4.7"
June	70	33	1.60"	0.4"
July	75	37	2.06"	0.0"
Aug.	74	36	2.08"	0.0"
Sept.	67	29	1.64"	1.1"
Oct.	57	22	1.28"	5.9"
Nov.	40	12	1.33"	18.9"
Dec.	32	3	1.66"	27.5"

Summer (June, July, August)

Expect sunny mornings; afternoon thunderstorms, accompanied by lightning. Nights are clear and cool.

Fall (September, October, November)

Expect mornings with frost; pleasant, clear afternoons; chilly nights. There is a possibility of early snowstorms.

Winter (December, January, February, March)

Expect cool to supercold mornings; high winds, blizzard conditions, and large temperature fluctuations.

Spring (April, May)

Temperatures are unpredictable at best; expect deep, wet snowfalls.

All seasons get a healthy helping of Colorado sunshine.

Altitude Sickness

Nothing ruins an outing more often than the body's resistance to altitude adjustment. The illness is usually characterized by vomiting, shortness of breath, extreme headache, lightheadedness, sleeplessness, and an overall sick feeling. Our advice: take it easy. When traveling to a higher altitude, give your body a day or two to adjust to less oxygen, hotter sun, and less air pressure. Drink plenty of water, and lay off the alcohol and cigarettes. Wear sunglasses and sunscreen. It's that easy. (As always, if serious symptoms persist, locate the nearest emergency room or call 911.)

Lightning

Get an early start on all hikes that go above tree line. Violent storms are common in June, July, and August. Try to reach high-altitude summits by 1 p.m. and turn back when the weather turns bad. If you get caught in a lightning storm above tree line, stay off ridgetops, spread out if you are in a group, and squat or sit on a foam pad with your feet together. Keep away from rock outcroppings and isolated trees. If someone has been struck, be prepared to use CPR to help restore breathing and heartbeat.

Hypothermia

Hypothermia occurs when your core body temperature is dangerously low. This condition can occur at any time of the year, and cold temperatures, wind, and rain and snow set the stage for complications. Look for signs of shivering, loss of coordination, and loss of judgment. Prevention in the form of preparation is your best defense against getting cold to the core. Remember the mantra "wet is not warm" to prevent hypothermia. Keep your inside layer as dry as possible.

CORSAR

The Colorado Outdoor Recreation Search and Rescue Card (CORSAR) may be purchased at most outdoor shops, such as REI. You can buy a one-year card for $3 or spend $12 and buy a five-year card. CORSAR is not insurance—it does not pay for medical transportation, which may include helicopter flights or ground ambulance. The card does allow reimbursement to county sheriffs for costs included on a mission.

These expenses can include mileage, meals, equipment, gasoline, and rental fees (horses, ATVs, aircraft) for vehicles used in the search. It says right on the CORSAR information that "you have helped ensure that trained and well-equipped search and rescue teams will respond should you become lost or in need of rescue and they will not have to incur undue expense due to your emergency."

Avalanches

When in snow-packed backcountry, avoid steep slopes and gullies where avalanches occur. Open slopes of 30 to 45 degrees can be loaded with dangerous masses of snow, easily triggered by the presence of one or more travelers. Check at the visitor centers for current snow conditions.

Swift Water

Mountain streams can be dangerous during high snow runoff in May and June. Even a narrow stream may be deep and fast, as well as cold. Remain back from the banks of streams and rivers, especially if you cannot see the bottom. Provide proper supervision for children who tend to be attracted to water. Rocks at the streamside and in the stream are often slippery, and water beneath them may be deep. Powerful currents in park streams can pull a person under water and pin him or her below the surface. In case of a flash flood, climb to safety.

Water

How much is enough? Well, one simple physiological fact should convince you to err on the side of excess when deciding how much water to pack: A hiker working hard in 90-degree heat needs about ten quarts of fluid per day. That's 2.5 gallons—12 large water bottles or 16 small ones. So pack along one or two bottles even for short hikes.

Some hikers and backpackers hit the trail prepared to purify water found along the route. This method, while less dangerous than drinking it untreated, comes with risks. Purifiers with ceramic filters are the safest. Many hikers pack along the slightly distasteful tetraglycine–hydroperiodide tablets to debug water (sold under the names Potable Aqua, Coughlan's, and others).

Probably the most common waterborne "bug" that hikers face is giardia, which may not hit until one to four weeks after ingestion. It will have you living in the bathroom, passing noxious rotten-egg gas, vomiting, and shivering with chills. Other parasites to worry about include E coli and cryptosporidium, both of which are harder to kill than giardia.

For most people, the pleasures of hiking make carrying water a relatively minor price to pay to remain healthy. If you're tempted to drink "found water," do so only if you understand the risks involved. Better yet, hydrate prior to your hike, carry (and drink) six ounces of water for every mile you plan to hike, and hydrate after the hike.

The Ten Essentials

See Appendix A: Camping-equipment Checklist (page 169) for a
comprehensive summer backpacking-gear checklist.

One of the first rules of hiking is to be prepared for anything.
The simplest way to be prepared is to carry the "Ten Essentials." In
addition to carrying the items listed below, you need to know how
to use them, especially navigation items. Always consider worst-case
scenarios like getting lost, hiking back in the dark, broken gear (for
example, a broken hip strap on your pack or a water filter getting
plugged), twisting an ankle, or a brutal thunderstorm. The items
listed below don't cost a lot of money, don't take up much room in
a pack, and don't weigh much, but they might just save your life.

WATER: durable bottles, and water treatment such as iodine
  or a filter

MAP: preferably a topo map and a trail map with a route description

COMPASS: a high-quality compass

FIRST-AID KIT: a good-quality kit, including first-aid instructions

KNIFE: a multitool device with pliers is best

LIGHT: flashlight or headlamp with extra bulbs and batteries

FIRE: windproof matches or lighter and fire starter

EXTRA FOOD: you should always have food in your pack when you've
  finished hiking

EXTRA CLOTHES: rain protection, warm layers, gloves, warm hat

SUN PROTECTION: sunglasses, lip balm, sunblock, sun hat

First-aid Kit

A typical first-aid kit may contain more items than you might
think necessary. The ones in the list that follows are just the basics.
Prepackaged kits in waterproof bags (Atwater Carey and Adventure

Medical make a variety of kits) are available. Even though quite a few items are listed below, they pack down into a small space:

Ace bandages or Spenco joint wraps

Antibiotic ointment (Neosporin or the generic equivalent)

Ibuprofen or acetaminophen

Band-Aids

Benadryl or the generic equivalent, diphenhydramine (in case of allergic reactions)

Butterfly-closure bandages

Epinephrine in a prefilled syringe (for severe allergic reactions to such things as bee stings; usually available by prescription only)

Gauze (one roll)

Gauze compress pads (a half-dozen 4- x 4-inch pads)

Hydrogen peroxide or iodine

Insect repellent

Matches or pocket lighter

Moleskin or Spenco "Second Skin"

Sunscreen

Whistle (it's more effective in signaling rescuers than your voice)

The following items are optional but worth their weight:

Aluminum foil

Bandana

Carabineers

Cellular phone (emergencies only)

Dark chocolate (at least 60 percent cocoa)

Digital camera

Disinfectant wipes (baby wipes)

Extra batteries

Flashlight

Foam pad (for lightning strikes)

Garbage bag

Gloves (for warmth)

GPS receiver

Hand warmers (air activated)

High-energy food and drinks

Lip balm

Long pants

Plastic bags with zip closure

Rain coat and rain pants

Shorts

Socks

Snakebite kit

Sunglasses

Toilet paper

Watch

Kim's Tips for Hiking and Camping with Children

Bringing your kids to Rocky Mountain National Park can be a great way to introduce the young to nature. It's also wonderful exercise and an even better family-bonding experience. It's time away from laundry, cell phones, and dishes—just you and the kids and nature.

PLANNING AND PACING

It's not advisable to take newborns out in the wild, but short walks in a stroller or a baby carrier are wonderful sensory and bonding opportunities. When my babies cried, I'd walk around our yard and point out leaves, trees, flowers, and birds. It calmed them and was a great way to build up to longer jaunts.

For children up to age 2, plan to pick them up or strap them in. Baby backpacks, baby carriers, strollers, bike trailers, and more all provide baby and parent with ample opportunity to get on the trail. Paved trails and well-maintained gravel trails all provide access to the younger set.

Children ages 2 to 4 can usually hike up to 2 miles. Be sure to plan plenty of extra time and know that you may end up carrying them. Children 5 to 7 can hike 3 to 4 miles over easy terrain. Resting, stopping, and plenty of wandering should be allowed for these age groups. Above age 8, children can easily hike a full day at a slow pace. A full day may include covering 6 miles over variable terrain. Set your entire group or family hiking goals based on the youngest child's ability. Preteens and teenagers may begin to hike more difficult trails if they have had hiking experience.

Children should be taught from the get-go that they must stay within eyesight of an adult. They are never to run off. Not only can they get lost or injured, but they can also cause damage to the trail or the ecosystem. Teach your kids to treat the outdoors kindly, and the outdoors will repay the favor.

Also teach your children to stay where they are if they do end up getting lost. Many children relate to hugging a tree when lost—instruct them to find one, hold on to it, and blow their whistle. Three whistle blows is the standard distress signal, which indicates, "I am lost" or "I need help." Likewise, never let kids go close to steep cliffs and other drop-off areas. Rules about going near rivers and other water sources and climbing on accessible rocks must be addressed as well. (My rule with my kids is "No!")

Always teach trail etiquette: leave no trace, pick up after others who do not, the uphill hiker has the right of way, and don't pick or pull anything. And of course, leaves of three, let them be.

Before you leave home, have the kids help make a special kid-friendly map of the area that they can keep in their bag. Making maps helps teach direction and creativity. Create a kid-friendly legend that has items such as waterfalls, trails, trees, or tents. Have the child mark interesting points of interest while they are hiking or camping.

Draw the route and have the child mark interesting waypoints while they are hiking.

Toy stores are home to many camping or backyard-camping things such as kids' magnifying glasses. A magnifying glass can be used to identify plants, insects, minerals in rocks, and flowers.

Make scavenger-hunt cards to use on any hike away from the campground (or in the area around the campground). A stack of index cards works fine. Have your child cut hiking-related items from used magazines and paste them on each card. If your child can draw, this works as well. Write the name under the item and bring as many as you want. You can prolong your scavenger hunt cards throughout the summer by simply marking each item that you see on the back. It's fun to have a trump card that could be tucked away for special sightings: bull snake, lost watch, or an abandoned sock. Bring a permanent marker to take notes on your cards—some may even want to laminate their cards.

Play games such as "I Spy," try bird-watching, look for animal tracks, or simply count rocks as you hike. The key is to play games that encourage children to observe their surroundings.

Assign a hiking leader (or mountain leader, as we call it), and have that child guide the hike. Plan on taking a lot of breaks, and at each break change the hiking leader.

Have your child invite a friend, which helps your child see the world from another youngster's perspective.

If the hike is going well, be sure to head home a little early, especially if you have to turn around and trace your steps. It is always better to end early on a positive note than to end with sore feet, a lot of whining, and discouraged hikers.

PACKING

Packing for the kids is much like packing for the parents. Be sure each camper-hiker has the U.S. Forest Service's "ten essentials": map, compass, water, knife, waterproof matches, high-energy food, suitable extra clothing (such as rain gear), mirror, first-aid kit, and whistle. Mom and Dad may want to carry the bulk of the weight and carry obvious things like the knife and matches. However, as kids can carry more, they will enjoy the responsibility, and parents don't end up schlepping it all around.

When hiking with a stroller or other apparatus, it's easy to stash extra essentials such as diapers and baby wipes. Consider packing my list of additional "ten kid essentials" for the trail: your child's favorite wholesome snack, juice, sunglasses, sunscreen, baby wipes, kid's trail map, kids' magnifying glass, scavenger hunt cards, lunch, and permanent markers.

Be sure everyone is dressed for the weather. For hot or cold days, the rule is to dress in layers. Start out with more in the winter and less in the summer. All children need to have one proper pair of socks and one proper pair of shoes. Be sure there is no cotton in the socks, since cotton retains moisture and helps create blisters. Instead, buy child-sized wool socks and nylon liners. Good tennis shoes are great, and child-sized hiking boots are even better.

For overnight hikes, each child needs a sleeping bag that will fit his or her body type and provide warmth. Do your research on sizes and temperature ratings. (Don't cave in and get the Barbie sleeping bag little Susie really wants. Save that for slumber parties indoors.)

ROCKY MOUNTAIN NATIONAL PARK'S COMMITMENT TO KIDS

Rocky Mountain National Park offers fabulous junior-ranger and ranger-led programs all year. Free junior-ranger books are available at park visitor centers for kids ages 6 to 12. A successfully completed book earns a badge.

General Safety

· **DO NOT EVER RELY ON CELL PHONES IN THE ROCKIES.** Signals and access are very inconsistent. Check with your cellular service provider before leaving home. Many outdoor enthusiasts rely on GPS and other forms of communication in the backcountry.

· **ALWAYS CARRY FOOD AND WATER** whether you are planning to go overnight or not. Food will give you energy, help keep you warm, and sustain you in an emergency situation until help arrives. You never know if you will have a stream nearby when you become thirsty. Bring potable water or treat water before drinking it from a stream. Boil or filter all found water before drinking it.

· **STAY ON DESIGNATED TRAILS.** Most hikers get lost when they leave the path. Even on the most clearly marked trails, there is usually a point where you have to stop and consider which direction to head. If you become disoriented, don't panic. As soon as you think you may be off track, stop, assess your current direction, and then retrace your steps back to the point where you went awry. Using a map, compass, this book, and keeping in mind what you have passed thus far, reorient yourself, and trust your judgment on which way to continue. If you become absolutely unsure of how to continue, return to your vehicle the way you came in. Should you become completely lost and have no idea of how to return to the trailhead, remaining in place along the trail and waiting for help is most often the best option for adults and always the best option for children.

· **BE ESPECIALLY CAREFUL WHEN YOU'RE CROSSING STREAMS.** Whether you are fording the stream or crossing on a log, make every step count. If you have any doubt about maintaining your balance on a foot log, go ahead and ford the stream instead. When fording a stream, use a trekking pole or stout stick for balance and face upstream as you cross. If a stream seems too deep to ford, turn back. Whatever is on the other side is not worth risking your life.

· **BE CAREFUL AT OVERLOOKS.** While these areas may provide spectacular views, they are potentially hazardous. Stay back from the edge of outcrops and be absolutely sure of your footing; a misstep can mean a nasty and possibly fatal fall.

- STANDING DEAD TREES and storm-damaged living trees pose a real hazard to hikers and tent campers. These trees may have loose or broken limbs that could fall at any time. When choosing a spot to rest or a backcountry campsite, look up.

- TAKE ALONG YOUR BRAIN. A cool, calculating mind is the single most important piece of equipment you'll ever need on the trail. Think before you act. Watch your step. Plan ahead. Avoiding accidents before they happen is the best recipe for a rewarding and relaxing hike.

- ASK QUESTIONS. Rocky Mountain National Park employees are there to help. It's a lot easier to gain advice beforehand and avoid a mishap away from civilization when it's too late to amend an error. Use your head out there and treat the place as if it were your own backyard. After all, it's your national park.

Animal and Plant Hazards

Rocky Mountain National Park has all sorts of wildlife: mule deer, bighorn sheep, coyote, elk, pika, moose, marmots, and more. Here's a quick primer on how best to enjoy watching wildlife:

- Never, ever feed wildlife.
- Watch from a distance.
- Obey all closure signs.
- Wildlife calls and spotlights are illegal in Rocky Mountain National Park.
- Drive cautiously and do not block traffic to look at wildlife.

BLACK BEARS

There are no definite rules about what to do if you meet a bear. In most cases the bear will detect you first and leave. If you do encounter a bear, here are some suggestions from the National Park Service:

- Stay calm.
- Move away, talking loudly to let the bear discover your presence.

- Back away while facing the bear.
- Avoid eye contact.
- Give the bear plenty of room to escape; bears will rarely attack unless they are threatened or provoked.
- Don't run or make sudden movements; running will provoke the bear, and you cannot outrun it.
- Do not attempt to climb trees to escape bears, especially black bears. The animal will pull you down by the foot.
- Fight back if attacked. Black bears have been driven away when people have fought back with rocks, sticks, binoculars, and even their bare hands.
- Be grateful that it's not a grizzly bear. There are none in Rocky Mountain National Park.

Mountain Lions

Lion attacks on people are rare, with fewer than 12 fatalities in 100 years. Based on observations by people who have come in contact with mountain lions, some patterns are beginning to emerge. Below are more suggestions from the National Park Service:

- Stay calm.
- Talk firmly to the lion.
- Move slowly.
- Back up or stop; never run because lions will chase and attack.
- Raise your arms. If you are wearing a sweater or coat; open it and hold it wide.
- Pick up children and make them appear larger.
- If the lion becomes aggressive, throw rocks and large objects at it. This is the time to convince the lion that you are not prey and that you are a danger to it.
- Never crouch down or turn your back to retrieve said items.
- Fight back and try to remain standing if you are attacked.

Ticks

Ticks like to hang out in the brush that grows along trails. Hot summer months seem to explode their numbers, but you should be tick-aware during all months of the year. Ticks, which are arthropods and not insects, need a host to feast on in order to reproduce. The ticks that light onto you while hiking will be very small, sometimes so tiny that you won't be able to spot them. Primarily of two varieties, deer ticks and dog ticks, both need a few hours of actual attachment before they can transmit any disease they may harbor. Ticks may settle in shoes, socks, hats, and may take several hours to actually latch on. The best strategy is to visually check every half-hour or so while hiking, do a thorough check before you get in the car, and then, when you take a post-hike shower, do an even more thorough check of your entire body. Ticks that haven't attached are easily removed, but not easily killed. If you pick off a tick in the woods, just toss it aside. If you find one on your body at home, dispatch it and then send it down the toilet. For ticks that have embedded, removal with tweezers is best.

Snakes

Rocky Mountain National Park is proud to claim that there is only one reptile species inside the park. It's the harmless garter snake. In any

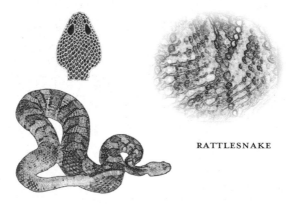

RATTLESNAKE

18

case, I like to include information on the venomous snake that is found in areas that border the park region. Rattler sightings are very common there, so why wouldn't one sneak across? A good rule of thumb is to give rattlers a wide berth and leave them alone. In the chance that you are bitten by a rattlesnake, stay calm and get help immediately.

On a side note, my husband was bitten by a rattlesnake in 1999. He was hiking alone and felt a slap on his leg. Luckily, hikers found him and a search-and-rescue team was deployed. He obviously survived!

Poison Ivy

Recognizing poison ivy and avoiding contact with it is the most effective way to prevent the painful, itchy rashes associated with this plant. Urushiol, the oil in the sap of poison ivy, is responsible for the rash. Usually within 12 to 14 hours of exposure (but sometimes much later), raised lines and/or blisters will appear, accompanied by a terrible itch. Refrain from scratching because bacteria under fingernails can cause infection and you will spread the rash to other parts of your body. Wash and dry the rash thoroughly, applying calamine lotion or another product to help dry the rash. If itching or blistering is severe, seek medical attention. Remember that oil-contaminated clothes, pets, or hiking gear can easily cause an irritating rash on you or someone else, so wash not only any exposed parts of your body but also clothes, gear, and pets.

COMMON POISONOUS PLANTS

POISON
SUMAC

POISON
OAK

POISON
IVY

MOSQUITOES

Although it's not a common occurrence, individuals can become infected with the West Nile virus by being bitten by an infected mosquito. Culex mosquitoes, the primary varieties that can transmit West Nile virus to humans, thrive in urban rather than natural areas. They lay their eggs in stagnant water and can breed in any standing water that remains for more than five days. Most people infected with West Nile virus have no symptoms of illness, but some may become ill, usually 3 to 15 days after being bitten.

In the park area, late spring and summer are the times thought to be the highest risk periods for mosquito bites and the possibility of the West Nile virus. At this time of year—and anytime you expect mosquitoes to be buzzing around—you may want to wear protective clothing, such as long sleeves, long pants, and socks. Loose-fitting, light-colored clothing is best. Spray clothing with insect repellent. Remember to follow the instructions on the repellent and to take extra care with children.

Tips for Enjoying Rocky Mountain National Park

- BEFORE YOU GO, visit the Rocky Mountain National Park Web site at **www.nps.gov/romo,** or call the park for an information kit at (970) 586-1206. Both resources will help you get oriented to Rocky Mountain National Park.

- MOST VISITORS ARRIVE DURING THE SUMMER MONTHS. Expect a lot of company on the roads, on some of the trails, and in the parking areas, especially between Memorial Day and Labor Day.

- ELEVATION IS AN INTEGRAL PART OF THE PARK EXPE- RIENCE. Don't push your physical limits in this region located above 8,000 feet. Altitude-sickness symptoms include shortness of breath, fatigue, dizziness, nausea, rapid heartbeat, and insomnia.

- **UPON ARRIVAL,** stop by a park visitor center for current information on everything from road and weather conditions to ranger-led programs.

- **THERE IS NO LODGING AVAILABLE INSIDE THE PARK,** but hundreds of accommodations are nearby in and around Estes Park and Grand Lake.

- **PETS ARE NOT PERMITTED** on any hiking trails.

- **BIKES ARE NOT PERMITTED** on any hiking trails.

- **A VALID COLORADO FISHING LICENSE** is required for fishing in the park. Annual, five-day and one-day resident and nonresident licenses are available. Licenses are sold at most sporting good stores.

- **THE PARK IS ALWAYS OPEN,** 24 hours a day all year.

- **ENTRANCE FEES:**
  Annual Pass: $35
  Seven-day automobile pass for individuals and families: $20
  America the Beautiful National Park and Federal Recreational Lands Pass: $80
  America the Beautiful Lifetime Senior Pass: $10 (age 62 and older)
  America the Beautiful Lifetime Access Pass: free (blind or permanently disabled)

- **TRAIL RIDGE ROAD USUALLY** opens for the season on Friday of Memorial Day weekend. Heavy snows typically close the road for the winter in mid- to late October.

- **OLD FALL RIVER ROAD IS USUALLY** open from early July to late September.

- **BEAR LAKE ROAD IS OPEN ALL YEAR,** but the park urges visitors to take advantage of the Bear Lake corridor shuttle bus available May 1 to October 10.

Tips for a Happy Camping Trip

There's nothing worse than a bad camping trip, especially since it's so easy to have a great time. To assist with making your outing a happy one, here are some pointers.

Always strive to practice low-impact camping. Adhere to the adages "Pack it in, pack it out," and "Take only pictures, leave only footprints." Practice "Leave No Trace" camping ethics while in the backcountry.

- **RESERVE YOUR SITE AHEAD OF TIME.** Permits are required for camping in the park's 269 designated backcountry campsites. See the extensive backcountry regulations in Appendix B: Rocky Mountain National Park Backcountry Camping Guide, on page 171. There are also five large campground neighborhoods found in the park: Aspenglen, Glacier Basin, Longs Peak, Moraine Park, and Timber Creek. For more information see the park's Web site (**www.nps.gov/romo**).

- **PICK YOUR CAMPING BUDDIES WISELY.** A family trip is pretty straightforward, but you may want to consider excluding grumpy Uncle Fred who doesn't like bugs, sunshine, or marshmallows. After you know who is going, make sure that everyone is on the same page regarding expectations of difficulty, sleeping arrangements, and food requirements.

- **DON'T DUPLICATE EQUIPMENT** such as cooking pots and lanterns among campers in your party. Carry what you need to have a good time, but don't turn the trip into a major moving experience.

- **DRESS APPROPRIATELY FOR THE SEASON.** Educate yourself on the highs and lows of the specific area you plan to visit. It may be warm at night in the summer in your backyard, but up in the mountains it will be quite chilly.

- **PITCH YOUR TENT ON A LEVEL SURFACE,** preferably one that is covered with leaves, pine straw, or grass. Pitch your tent on a tarp or specially designed footprint to thwart ground moisture and to protect the tent floor. Do a little site maintenance such as picking up small rocks and sticks that can damage your tent floor and make sleep uncomfortable. If you have a separate tent rain fly but don't need it, keep it rolled up at the base of the tent in case it starts raining at midnight.

- **TAKE A SLEEPING PAD WITH YOU.** Use one that is full-length and thicker than you think you might need. This will not only keep your hips from aching on hard ground, but will also help keep you warm.

- **IF YOU ARE NOT HIKING INTO A PRIMITIVE CAMPSITE,** there is no real need to skimp on food due to weight. Plan tasty meals and bring everything you will need to prepare, cook, eat, and clean up the mess.

- **IF YOU'RE PRONE TO USING THE BATHROOM MULTIPLE TIMES AT NIGHT,** you should plan ahead. Leaving a warm sleeping bag and stumbling around in the dark to find the restroom, whether it be an outhouse, a fully plumbed facility, or just the woods, is second best. Keep a flashlight and any other accoutrements you may need by the tent door and know exactly where to head in the dark.

- **STANDING DEAD TREES** and storm-damaged living trees can pose a real hazard to tent campers. These trees may have loose or broken limbs that could fall at any time. When choosing a spot to rest or a backcountry campsite, look up.

Trail and Camping Etiquette

Always remember that great care and resources (from nature as well as from your tax dollars) have gone into creating these trails. Treat the trail, wildlife, and fellow hikers with respect.

- **HIKE ON OPEN TRAILS ONLY.**

- **LEAVE ONLY FOOTPRINTS.** Be sensitive to the ground beneath you. This also means staying on the existing trail and not blazing any new trails. Be sure to pack out what you pack in. No one likes to see the trash someone else has left behind.

- **NEVER SPOOK ANIMALS.** An unannounced approach, a sudden movement, or a loud noise startles most animals. A surprised moose can be dangerous to you, to others, and to themselves. Give animals extra room and time to adjust to your presence.

- **PLAN AHEAD.** Know your equipment, your ability, and the area where you are hiking—and prepare accordingly. Be self-sufficient at all times; carry necessary supplies for changes in weather or other conditions. A well-executed trip is a satisfaction to you and to others.

- **BE COURTEOUS TO OTHER** hikers or equestrians you meet on the trails.

- **OBTAIN ALL PERMITS AND AUTHORIZATION AS REQUIRED.** Make sure you check in, pay your fee, and mark your site as directed. Don't make the mistake of grabbing a seemingly empty site that looks more appealing than your site. It could be reserved.

- **FOLLOW THE PARK'S RULES REGARDING THE BUILDING OF FIRES.** It's firmly discouraged and against regulations at most campsites.

Northeast Side of Rocky Mountain National Park

NORTH FORK AREA AND MUMMY RANGE

1

More
than 110
mountain
peaks
tower
over
the 415
square
miles of
hiking
trails
picnic
spots
waterfalls
cold lakes
and
bountiful
wildlife

01 Cow Creek Trailhead: *Bridal Veil Falls*

SCENERY: ☆ ☆ ☆ ☆	DISTANCE: *6.44 miles out-and-back*
TRAIL CONDITION: ☆ ☆ ☆ ☆	HIKING TIME: *3.5 hours*
CHILDREN: ☆ ☆ ☆	OUTSTANDING FEATURES: *Thundering*
DIFFICULTY: ☆ ☆ ☆	*waterfall; meadow and alpine landscape;*
SOLITUDE: ☆ ☆ ☆	*historical ranch*

A gentle trail gives way to a strenuous push on the last portion of this uncrowded, undiscovered beauty. More like a bridezilla than a bride, the Bridal Veil Falls crash into Cow Creek, plummeting more than 20 vertical feet from a broken rock face—the tallest falls in the park. Spring is the best time of year to visit the falls since the recent snowmelt contributes to the falls torrent. The shoulder seasons are also nice since this is a sunny hike that can be quite warm in the summer.

🏃 From Cow Creek Trailhead at McGraw Ranch, hike west along Cow Creek Trail, which begins as a level, dirt access road. Hikers enter the ranch on foot, passing over Cow Creek, up the drive, and through the side of the ranch gate. Pass Indian Head Ranch, which is better known as Old McGraw Ranch, on the left. Pioneered and homesteaded in the 1870s, the property was later used as a cattle ranch and then as a guest ranch. The buildings, which are owned by the National Park Service, are in current use as a research and learning center accessed by universities and educational groups.

Just beyond McGraw Ranch is the junction of Cow Creek Trail with the North Boundary Trail. The rustic Forest Service–looking buildings are small in comparison to the large rock formations known as Lumpy Ridge that dominate this area. A glasslike pond, bordered by a mountain meadow, completes the unique beginnings of this trail.

01 Cow Creek Trailhead: **Bridal Veil Falls**

0   1,500   3,000
feet

ROOSEVELT
NATIONAL FOREST

West Creek

McGraw Ranch Rd.

N. Boundary Trl.

COMANCHE PEAK
WILDERNESS

Gem Lake Trl.

Cow Creek Trl.

Cow Creek

ROCKY MTN.
NATIONAL PARK

horse hitch

Bridal Veil
Falls

To 34

Continue along Cow Creek Trail, through the open meadow, pass a restroom, and head toward the pine forest for 1.2 miles. Cross through the significant intersection of Cow Creek Trail, Bridal Veil Falls, Lawn Lake, Balance Rock, Gem Lake, and Twin Owls Parking. Take the right fork and continue straight on Cow Creek Trail toward Bridal Veil Falls, which is 2 miles from this point. Lawn Lake, another popular destination from this trailhead, is 8.1 miles. The trail is flanked by meadows on either side with mountains on either side of each meadow. Pine trees, spring flowers, and the sound of humming birds dominated our hike in late spring.

The trail is now a single-track and has narrowed from the wide road. Hikers can no longer walk side by side. The trail gently ascends and Cow Creek drops to the left. After another 0.2 miles, pass the turn off to Rabbit Ears Campsite on the left. Above the trail, the rock formation illustrates its nomenclature. The site is located in a secluded, shaded area near Cow Creek and is available to a small group by backcountry permit only.

The trail continues west and joins Cow Creek once again, traveling along its edge. Sheep Mountain overlooks Cow Creek and the north side of Lumpy Ridge. Its sheer south face is sometimes visited by technical rock climbers. At approximately 2 miles from the trailhead, arrive at another trail intersection with Cow Creek Trail, Bridal Veil Falls, Black Canyon Trail, and Lawn Lake Trail. Head right as the trail exits the meadow and begins a more gradual ascent into the forest.

The trail gets steeper and for the last section, hikers cross over Cow Creek a few times via man-made bridges. The forest becomes dense and the trail becomes narrow and rocky. The next trail waypoint is a hitch rack for horses, which signifies that the last portion of the trail is inaccessible to them. Hikers will see why as they traverse over steep rock slabs and into a narrow gorge. The trail is not marked well from this point, so pay attention to your footing, the foot path, and the cairns that signify turns in the trail. The sound from the falls will also be your guide. As it gets louder and the creek becomes wilder, you will be getting closer.

After climbing a set of man-made stone steps, hikers arrive at the Bridal Veil Falls. The obvious name choice for this distinctive water formation creates the illusion of a bride's mysterious, gauzy, flowing hair piece. The thundering water hitting the base of rocks and sending a spray of mist is always a crowd-pleaser—especially if the only crowd is your hiking group. Hike above the falls if you want to see the upper part of the falls and a close-up of the steep wall that forms the main section of the falls. Find a nice picnic spot, rest, then turn around and travel back to the trailhead the way that you came.

DIRECTIONS: From Estes Park, take US 34 until it intersects Big Thompson Avenue/Elkhorn Avenue and turns into Wonderview Avenue. Pass the Stanley Historic District and take the first right onto MacGregor Avenue. Travel 3.5 miles from MacGregor Ranch Road, and then take a left at McGraw Ranch Road. Continue for 2.5 miles to the trailhead; parallel park in designated areas only.

GPS Trailhead Coordinates	01 COW CREEK TRAILHEAD: BRIDAL VEIL FALLS
UTM zone (WGS84):	13T
Easting:	0457590
Northing:	4475500

Happily Lost Campsite

SCENERY: ✰ ✰ ✰ ✰	DISTANCE: *12.5 miles out–and–back*
TRAIL CONDITION: ✰ ✰	HIKING TIME: *7 hours*
CHILDREN: ✰	OUTSTANDING FEATURES: *Remote, lesser*
DIFFICULTY: ✰ ✰ ✰ ✰	*used part of the park, dense forest, follows river most*
SOLITUDE: ✰ ✰ ✰ ✰ ✰	*of the way, soft trail*

The trail to Happily Lost is unique to this book. Like its namesake, the trail leaves you feeling lost in the wilderness: remoteness, variety, and density define the experience. This is a great trail for a hot summer day. The campsite is very private and very hidden. The forest is so dense here that we cannot say enough about its "Black Forest" appeal. After the first mile, you do cross through civilization at Camp Cheley, but it passes quickly.

🚶🚶 Leave the trailhead and follow the North Fork Trail as it travels up a short rise and then begins a sharp descent to the North Fork of the Big Thompson River. At the sign directing hikers toward Rocky Mountain National Park, take a right turn. Hike along the river while noting spots to stop and cool your feet on the return trip. There are a lot of pools and eddies in this first leg of the North Fork. The trail is narrow along the river.

Hike up the ravine where the trail is lush, green, and seemingly in its own world. Begin to cross a series of large wooden bridges that cross back and forth across the North Fork. Approach what looks like a large luxury log home, but you will then see a horse corral, basketball court, and archery range. This is a branch of the famed Cheley Camp. In younger days I camped at their main lodges off Marys Lake Road.

Pass the horse shed and corral, cross the bridge, and start to leave the camp behind. The trail joins with a short stretch of narrow road

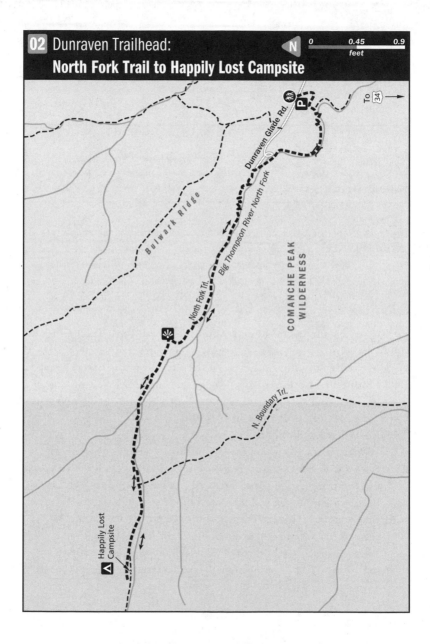

N

0   0.45   0.9
feet

To 34

Dunraven Glade Rd.

Bulwark Ridge

North Fork Trl.

Big Thompson River North Fork

COMANCHE PEAK WILDERNESS

N. Boundary Trl.

Happily Lost Campsite

that's part of the camp. The trail then turns to soft, deep sand, which requires a little more effort going up, but coming down, the sand feels nice on tired feet. Time for more bridges, and then the terrain opens up a little bit as the ravine widens to a valley. There is a view now, but it is slightly obscured by the lodgepole-pine forest. Continue to another bridge; before you cross it you will spot a Forest Service campsite. Do not confuse these sites with the Rocky Mountain National Park campsites. They are totally separate and sit in the Comanche Peak Wilderness. Pass another campsite after the bridge. The trail makes an abrupt change to a narrow, hard-packed-dirt path, but it doesn't last.

Cross through the meadow, lined with stately ponderosa pine trees. At this point, hikers will encounter a steeper trail. The second half of the trail has the most elevation gain.

Pass the remains of a cabin, left over from an old hunting resort, appropriately named Deserted Village. On the left are also more Forest Service campsites. Cross a small stream and continue across another meadow past Forest Service campsite #9.

After traveling in a straight line for some time, the trail has an uncharacteristic switchback. Head northeast and away from the water for a change. Pay attention to the trail because the path is steep and hard to follow. Stop at a nice resting spot on the rocks, complete with views.

Pass through the boundary to Rocky Mountain National Park. A higher standard of trail maintenance exists here and is evident from the start. The log stairs and erosion devices make it obvious. Rejoin the river at the small cascade on the left. Continue, passing a few campsites and the intersection with the North Boundary Trail. Enter a lichen-draped forest. Pass the Kettle Tarn Campsite and the Halfway Campsite. Halfway earned its namesake because it is located at half the elevation gain for those hiking to Lost Lake. At this point you've gained 1,400 feet from the trailhead. We continue another 0.9 miles and 200 feet of elevation to the Happily Lost Campsite. Go left into the campsite and follow the red marker signs into the dense forest. The trail winds to the right, and it is there that you spot the silver arrow that marks the designated campsite. Two small tent sites and a little fire pit are located 100 feet from the river. There are some views peeking out from the shelter of the forest. On the other side of the main trail is the privy. This campsite offers a deep-woods experience, situated in a cool, dark forest. Be sure to set up camp early and forego the scary campfire stories for the night. Have a nice rest, and in the morning, head back the way that you came.

DIRECTIONS: Take US 34 west from Loveland for 17 miles to Drake. Turn right on CR 43 and travel 6 miles to CR 518, past the Glen Haven Post Office and the sign that says FOREST ACCESS 2¼ MILES. Turn left onto the dirt road and drive 2.25 miles to the parking lot and trailhead.

GPS Trailhead Coordinates	02 DUNRAVEN TRAILHEAD: NORTH FORK TRAIL TO HAPPILY LOST CAMPSITE (OVERNIGHT)
UTM zone (WGS84):	13T
Easting:	0461010
Northing:	4480430

Upper Chipmunk Campsite

SCENERY: ✪ ✪ ✪ ✪
TRAIL CONDITION: ✪ ✪ ✪ ✪
CHILDREN: ✪ ✪
DIFFICULTY: ✪ ✪ ✪ ✪
SOLITUDE: ✪ ✪ ✪

DISTANCE: *8.4 miles out-and-back*
HIKING TIME: *5 hours*
OUTSTANDING FEATURES: *Horseshoe Falls, Chipmunk Lake, Ypsilon Mountain and Ypsilon Lake, forest, Roaring River*

This hike is full of drama: the Y-shaped, snow-filled scar on Ypsilon Mountain; Horseshoe Falls and the canyon gorged by the escaped dam waters of Lawn Lake; and the lung-busting climb of the Ypsilon Trail. You'll be widely entertained— not to mention sufficiently tired—at the end of this hike to the Upper Chipmunk Campsite, which is located between Chipmunk Lake and Ypsilon Lake and provides access to both.

🚶 Leave the trailhead and start on Lawn Lake Trail. Go up the man-made stairs and continue to the first major intersection of Ypsilon Lake, Lawn Lake, and Deer Mountain trails. Take a left turn here. The next junction is an intersection with a horse trail—stay straight. The trail travels at a slight ascent; it's sandy and full of rocks.

The hike continues with a series of switchbacks. After a half mile the trail passes along Horseshoe Falls and the Alluvial Fan of mud, sand, and boulders that swept down into Horseshoe Park when the 1982 Lawn Lake flood made its destructive path.

At the intersection of Ypsilon Lake and the Lawn Lake Trail, take a left turn following the Ypsilon Lake signs. The trail is very sandy and almost beachlike as it approaches the Roaring River. Cross the river on a split-log bridge. After the bridge, cross into the forest and begin the arduous trek uphill. It's an unforgiving hill that offers only a few restful switchbacks at the very end. The steepest areas are

N

0   1,500   3,000
feet

Upper Chipmunk Lake

Upper Chipmunk Campsites

Chipmunk Lake

Ypsilon Trl.

Lawn Lake Trl.

Roaring River

ROCKY MTN. NATIONAL PARK

Horseshoe Falls

Old Fall River Rd.

Endo Valley Rd.

Lawn Lake Trl.

Fall River

Thousand Falls

Alluvial Fan

34

secured by log steps, and the trail is lined on both sides by dense lodgepole-pine trees.

After climbing for the better part of 2.5 miles, the trail begins to level out and descend. Ahead are the first spectacular views of Ypsilon Mountain and her formidable, southeast facing couloir. A long 4 miles from the trailhead and the beginning of the hike, you pass the southwest side of Chipmunk Lake. It is a small alpine lake, lined by boulders and a marshy shore and framed by large lodgepole-pine trees. Pass a giant boulder field and take a right turn onto the Upper Chipmunk Campsite access trail.

The Upper Chipmunk Campsite is another 0.2 miles into the woods. You cannot see Chipmunk Lake from here, but there are tree-obscured views of Ypsilon Mountain and Ypsilon Lake. There are two designated campsites and a privy in the middle of the woods with no shelter. The sites are located in a dense pine forest on the edge of the Ypsilon Lake drainage. This is a great place to rest for the night or to just have a nice private picnic.

No trip to the Upper Chipmunk Campsite would be complete without a visit to the shore of Ypsilon Lake. Be sure to make a side trip down the trail as it descends sharply and then climbs a little, and then descends again to Ypsilon Lake. You will pass the waterfalls from neighboring lakes. The trail skirts the lake along most of its shore, except for the dramatic rise of Ypsilon Mountain on the northwest shore.

Whether camping, or hiking for the day, trace your way back to Chipmunk Lake and then head back the trailhead the way that you came.

DIRECTIONS: From the Beaver Meadows Entrance take US 36 west to the intersection of US 36 and US 34. Turn right onto US 34 and travel 1.8 miles to the turn for Old Fall River Road. Turn left onto Old Fall River Road, and then take a right into the Lawn Lake Trailhead parking lot.

GPS Trailhead Coordinates	03 LAWN LAKE TRAILHEAD: YPSILON TRAIL TO UPPER CHIPMUNK CAMPSITE (OVERNIGHT)
UTM zone (WGS84):	13T
Easting:	0446930
Northing:	4472930

SCENERY: ✩ ✩ ✩ ✩	DISTANCE: *3.4 miles out-and-back*
TRAIL CONDITION: ✩ ✩ ✩ ✩	HIKING TIME: *2.5 hours*
CHILDREN: ✩ ✩ ✩	OUTSTANDING FEATURES: *Views of Estes*
DIFFICULTY: ✩ ✩ ✩	*Park, Rocky Mountain National Park, Twin Owls,*
SOLITUDE: ✩ ✩ ✩	*alpine lake*

Gem Lake, if you'll pardon the pun, is a jewel. Located on the eastern edge of Rocky
Mountain National Park, this trailhead is one of the closest to the town of Estes Park.

To begin this hike, leave your car and walk to the trailhead
and signs that mark the beginning of the Gem Lake Trail. Gem
Lake's lower elevation in relation to the rest of Rocky Mountain
National Park, along with the hike's southern exposure, make this
a great year-round hike. Estes Park is home to retirees, families,
and other outdoors enthusiasts, so both the very old and very young
frequent this trail.

In 2007, the Twin Owls and Gem Lake trailheads were combined
and renamed the Lumpy Ridge Trailhead. Until then, the trails split
the crowds pretty evenly, so access to Gem Lake may be a little more
crowded than usual. You're also hiking a trail that is 0.3 miles shorter
than those I've featured in previous books.

In a few yards a steady climb begins, supplemented by short
switchbacks that weave in and out of the trees and skirt around large
rocks. After 0.5 miles, the Gem Lake Trail reaches a junction with the
trail that leads west to the Twin Owls—massive rock formations that
resemble two giant owls resting on the crest of the hill. This intersection mostly marks access for rock climbers and their left turn to the
owls, which you can see as you access the trailhead by car (a good point
of reference is to look behind the Stanley Hotel). The climbing here
is very technical, and climbers observe a strict code of conduct.

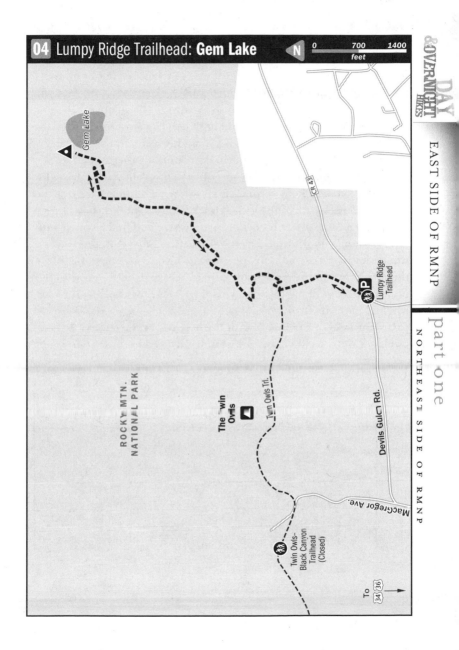

04 Lumpy Ridge Trailhead: **Gem Lake**

N

0   700   1400
feet

DAY
& OVERNIGHT
HIKES

EAST SIDE OF RMNP

part one
NORTHEAST SIDE OF RMNP

Gem Lake

CR 43

Lumpy Ridge Trailhead

ROCKY MTN.
NATIONAL PARK

The Twin
Owls

Twin Owls Trl.

Devils Gulch Rd.

MacGregor Ave.

Twin Owls–
Black Canyon
Trailhead
(Closed)

To
34 36

Staying on the Gem Lake Trail, turn right (east) and follow the trail as it climbs moderately. To the right, catch the first views of Rocky Mountain National Park and one of its more famous mountains: Longs Peak. A popular "fourteener," or peak 14,000 feet or higher, Longs can be found by looking for the silhouette of a beaver climbing up the side of a hill. The peak is at the beaver's nose.

Follow the sandy footpath near where heavy foot traffic has cut many random paths to scenic overlooks. Continue over smooth rock outcroppings and drink in the views of Lake Estes and Estes Park. The trail veers to the left and becomes even softer and sandier. On one of my hikes here, I saw a young racked buck, a rare sight this close to town.

Descend into a small, rocky canyon where you find a bench and Paul Bunyan's Boot. Another rock formation of legend, this one resembles an outsize boot propped on its heel. (Note the hole in the sole.) Continue up the many switchbacks, passing a precariously placed outhouse along the way. This portion of the trail is quite narrow and navigates through a large boulder field and granite slabs.

Gem Lake comes into view at the base of granite cliffs with boulders and a small beach at the water's edge. This mountain lake is a bit cold for the body, but a few minutes' respite here will cleanse the soul. When the sun hits the water, you'll see the mix of jewel tones—emerald, sapphire, ruby, and diamond—that gives the lake its name.

To return to the trailhead, head back the way you came. If you have more time, there are plenty of hikes that continue past Gem Lake and venture for hours, if not days, into Rocky Mountain National Park.

DIRECTIONS: From Estes Park, take US 34 until it intersects Big Thompson Avenue/Elkhorn Avenue and turns into Wonderview Avenue. Pass the Stanley Historic District and take the first right onto MacGregor Avenue. Follow MacGregor as it veers right and turns into Devils Gulch Road, and follow it until you reach the Lumpy Ridge Trailhead turnoff on the left.

GPS Trailhead Coordinates	04 LUMPY RIDGE TRAILHEAD: GEM LAKE
UTM zone (WGS84):	13T
Easting:	0456920
Northing:	4471410

East Center of Rocky Mountain National Park

Gorge Lakes Area and Bear Lake Area

2

More
than 11,0
mountai
peak
towe
ove
the 41
squar
miles o
hiking
trails
picni
spot
waterfalls
cold lakes
an
bountif
wildlif

SCENERY: ✿ ✿ ✿
TRAIL CONDITION: ✿ ✿ ✿ ✿
CHILDREN: ✿ ✿ ✿
DIFFICULTY: ✿ ✿
SOLITUDE: ✿ ✿

DISTANCE: *5 miles out–and–back*
HIKING TIME: *2.5 hours*
OUTSTANDING FEATURES: *Aspen trees, mountain lake*

Four main trails service Bierstadt Lake. Bear Lake Trailhead is an easier, longer option because the trailhead is slightly higher than the subalpine lake destination. So instead of heading up and away, you can treat yourself to a gradual descent with a worthy reward. The up part can come at the end this time.

From the Bear Lake Trailhead, follow the masses past the entrance to the Bear Lake hikes. Of all the paths at this trailhead, this one is the easiest to find—being a popular winter cross-country-skiing trail, it's marked with orange fluorescent squares.

From here, follow the Flattop Mountain Trail, which heads to Odessa Lake, for approximately 0.4 miles to the intersection of Bierstadt Lake Trail.

Bierstadt Lake was named after Albert Bierstadt, a famous 19th-century painter. He's most renowned for the large canvases that he sold to royalty, paintings portraying the West and the landscapes of the Rockies. One such depiction of Estes Park and Longs Peak was commissioned by the Earl of Dunraven, who took it to Europe to hang in the Dunraven Castle.

Continue straight toward Bierstadt Lake. The trail, up to this point is characterized by a small climb through the trees, both aspen and pine. As promised, the trail now descends along an easy, wooded path for 0.75 miles to the intersection of Bierstadt Lake Trial, Mill Creek Basin, and Hollowell Park. Continue straight.

N

0   1000   2000
feet

To
34 36

Mill Creek

Bierstadt
Lake

Bierstadt Lake Trl.

Bear Lake Rd.

Glacier Creek

Loch Trl.

Bear
Lake

Bear Lake
Trailhead

The next intersection is with the loop trail around Bierstadt Lake where hikers continue straight and begin a clockwise circle around the lake. Another intersection passes quickly and it is another meeting with Mill Creek Basin and Hollowell Park to the left. Keep heading to the right to complete your loop of the lake.

Picturesque Bierstadt Lake, offers fabulous views that stretch from Notchtop Mountain to Longs Peak. The optimal view of Longs Peak is from the north side of the lake. Due to thick tree cover, the lake is very rarely visible from the trail around it. Hikers must take various spurs or social trails to get to the lake's shore. There are a few small beaches perfect for a picnic or rest. The shallowest edges of the lake are filled with plant life that grows in and out of the water.

Continue heading right at the intersection with the Bierstadt Lake Trailhead trail. This trail is a shorter, more difficult hike that zigzags up 1.4 miles the south side of Bierstadt Moraine from the Bierstadt Lake Trailhead. One option, during the shuttle bus season, is to take the Bierstadt Lake Trail down to the Bierstadt Lake Trailhead on Bear Lake Road and take the shuttle bus back to your car a the Bear Lake Trailhead.

If you are going to stick to the original plan, when you get back to the beginning of the loop, turn left and head back the way you came to the Bear Lake Trailhead.

DIRECTIONS: From Estes Park go to Rocky Mountain National Park's Beaver Meadows Entrance Station via US 36. After entering the park, go 0.2 miles, take a left at Bear Lake Road, and travel 9.3 miles to the Bear Lake Trailhead parking lot.

GPS Trailhead Coordinates	05 BEAR LAKE TRAILHEAD: BIERSTADT LAKE
UTM zone (WGS84):	13T
Easting:	0445158
Northing:	4462391

SCENERY: ☆ ☆ ☆ ☆	DISTANCE: *3.6 miles out-and-back*
TRAIL CONDITION: ☆ ☆ ☆	HIKING TIME: *2 hours*
CHILDREN: ☆ ☆ ☆	OUTSTANDING FEATURES: *Three mountain*
DIFFICULTY: ☆ ☆ ☆	*lakes, alpine forest, variety of streams*
SOLITUDE: ☆	

Here you get three lakes for the price of one. Add in Bear Lake and that's four lakes for the price of one. The lakes are all unique and spaced apart nicely to keep hikers paced and interested. Because of the obvious value of this hike, it can be very crowded. Even in late spring, you'll traverse snow.

🚶 Leave Bear Lake Trailhead. At the trail mileage sign for Emerald Lake 1.8 miles, take a left turn. When we hiked in spring, the wide beginnings of this trail were packed with people. At the next fork, take a right turn, heading up the hill.

The trail is comprised of rough asphalt. Continue to travel at a slight ascent. The trail is framed by pine and aspen trees. Views of the mountain ranges are to your left and a hillside is immediately to the right.

Hiker's first destination, Nymph Lake, comes up quickly after 0.5 miles. In early June, snow still flanks its edges. The lake is deep, dark blue, and calm with only the pine forest reflected in its mirror. Lily pads float on its surface in the summer. The trail continues to head up and around the back of Nymph Lake. Cross through a boulder field, descend for a short time and then continue. The path is no longer asphalt and is instead a soft, dirt-packed single-track. In the summer, expect to cross through small streams and marshy spots full of mountain wildflowers. Flattop Mountain, Hallett Peak, and Longs Peak are all in view from the trail from one point or another. While the lakes share similar backdrops, they are all unique

52

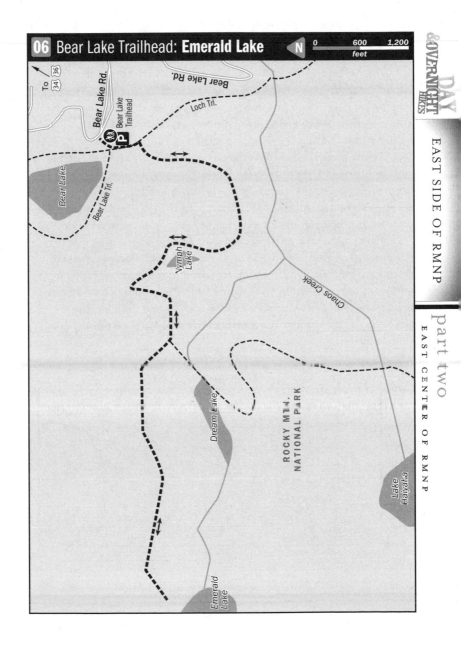

06 Bear Lake Trailhead: **Emerald Lake**

N

0   600   1,200
feet

To 34 36

Bear Lake Rd.

Bear Lake Rd.

Loch Trl.

Bear Lake Trailhead

P

Bear Lake

Bear Lake Trl.

Nymph Lake

Chaos Creek

Dream Lake

ROCKY MTN. NATIONAL PARK

Lake Haiyaha

Emerald Lake

and range from the lushness of Nymph Lake to the sereneness of Dream Lake to the drama of Emerald Lake.

The next stop is Dream Lake after the trail enters the forest and takes hikers through a few steep switchbacks. The open shores of Dream Lake seem to drink in and consume the surrounding forest and rock formations giving it an almost surreal or dreamlike quality—thus the name.

Continue around the lake, heading toward Emerald Lake. The trail to Emerald Lake follows the north shore of Dream Lake and then climbs over rocks before it levels out. Conditions at this point, especially when we hiked, were muddy and snow packed, which discouraged many of the crowds that subsequently turned back.

After passing the northwest edge of Dream Lake, continue to climb the trail along the banks of Tyndall Creek. The trail passes through the forest, continues up the man-made staircase along a waterfall. Surrounded by rock spires and talus slopes, Emerald Lake is truly a scenic destination. When we hiked in late spring, the tracks from backcountry snow riders were still visible from the lake's sloped shores.

Tyndall Gorge rises to the west and into the Continental Divide. From here you can also see the north face of Hallett Peak and the south side of Flattop Mountain. Steep rock walls on all sides, except for the side that hosts the trail, offer no escape—not that you need one! I thought we needed a quick escape when a tame chipmunk climbed my husband's back and gave me quite a scare when Bruce screamed for his life.

After a quick respite on one of the sun-baked boulders at the end of the trail, turn around and go back to the trailhead the same way you came.

DIRECTIONS: From Estes Park go to Rocky Mountain National Park's Beaver Meadows Entrance Station via US 36. After entering the park, go 0.2 miles, take a left at Bear Lake Road, and travel 9.3 miles to the Bear Lake Trailhead parking lot.

GPS Trailhead Coordinates	06 BEAR LAKE TRAILHEAD: EMERALD LAKE
UTM zone (WGS84):	13T
Easting:	0445158
Northing:	4462301

SCENERY: ✿ ✿ ✿ ✿ ✿	DISTANCE: *8.8 miles out-and-back*
TRAIL CONDITION: ✿ ✿ ✿ ✿	HIKING TIME: *6 hours (going approximately*
CHILDREN: ✿	*1.5 mph)*
DIFFICULTY: ✿ ✿ ✿ ✿ ✿	OUTSTANDING FEATURES: *Timberline, views*
SOLITUDE: ✿ ✿ ✿	*of alpine lakes, tundra, summit hike*

Flattop Mountain is a large, flat summit space that offers access to the Continental Divide and the trails that crisscross from Estes Park to Grand Lake. It is a well-known hike that many locals gasp at and grab their legs when talking of their last trip to Flattop. The trail is well-maintained even though it travels through timberline and alpine tundra. The crowds of Bear Lake disappear quickly as the long alpine climb (almost 3,000 feet elevation gain!) takes shape.

🚶🚶 From the Bear Lake parking lot follow the sign pointing hikers to Bear Lake along a nicely appointed trail, complete with railings lining the side. At the sign for Flattop Mountain, take a right turn and begin to head uphill. The trail is now unpaved and travels through a dense aspen grove above Bear Lake. This smooth hard-packed-dirt path is wide and very well maintained, and it starts a slight grade that will be commonplace, if not steeper for the next 4 miles. Continue to follow the signs to Flattop Mountain because a fork appears in the trail right away. The right turn goes to Bierstadt Lake. Continue on the trail, going left and still climbing.

A little less than a mile from Bear Lake is another major trail intersection. Continue in a hard left onto a steep switchback. The trail to the right goes to Odessa Lake and Fern Lake. The trail to Flattop Mountain continues to switchback in a zigzag pattern; traveling uphill in a very rocky, hard-packed part of the trail. The rockiness will be typical of the rest of the trail, and many hikers

0   1,350   2,700
feet

To 34 36

Bierstadt Lake Trl.

Bear Lake Rd.

The Loch Trl.

Glacier Gorge Jct.

P

Bear Lake

Bear Lake Trl.

Nymph Lake

Emerald Lake Trl.

Dream Lake

Lake Haiyaha

ROCKY MTN. NATIONAL PARK

Emerald Lake

Two Rivers Lake

Helene Lake

Grace Falls

Flattop Mtn.

Tyndall Glacier

at this point realize that they need to reevaluate the hike, find that they are not up to the elevation gain and grade, and turn around.

For the next 1.5 miles, several long switchbacks usher hikers up the steep terrain. They are so long that it's difficult to recognize the true nature of the switchback. They are not your customary swing-and-loop, back-and-forth switchbacks.

The trail takes you southwest, then back northwest, then back southwest again, and eventually hikers arrive at a very-well-marked Dream Lake overlook. Up to this point, Longs Peak has been prominent on the left side of the hike. Views of Mills Lake and the area across Glacier Gorge, the valley below Longs Peak, are prominent. The mountain that seems to come into view every now and then is also very visible here. It is the dramatic, angular Hallett Peak.

This completes the first half of the hike. It's characterized by a grade that is consistently unrelenting and uphill. The trail travels through pine, spruce, and fir trees with views popping up here and there on the switchbacks and in the trees.

Some hikes exit tree line abruptly; this one takes its time, with the trees slowly getting shorter and stunted—the twisted growth, also known as krummholz, sticks with you for a while. After a mile of these games, hikers will finally be past tree line and into the tundra. The miscellaneous switchbacks that have been crisscrossing all throughout the hike continue. The rocky terrain gets a little more challenging, and eventually hikers will come to a series of switchbacks where the last turn in the series rewards hikers with a tremendous and well-marked overlook of Emerald Lake far below. The sign says DO NOT DESCEND, but I don't think that's a problem since it's a looming 1,300 feet below. This is especially true if you are afraid of heights, as most of my hiking companions are. Take the warning seriously, since fatal accidents have occurred when blinding snowstorms and stumbling over a precipice have mixed. The area in view is also known as Tyndall Gorge. Longs Peak is prominent to your left, as well as during most of the time spent above tree line. You cannot see the Flattop Mountain summit—not yet.

Looking behind, you can see Sprague Lake, the road up toward Bear Lake, and sitting in a slight depression on top of a mountain a little closer is Bierstadt Lake. Scamper over rock piles arranged in various jumbles as you visualize little mountain pikas moving here and there across their native landscape. Just as energy follows thought, you will see what will most likely be your first pika. These active little creatures are characterized by round ears and a rabbitlike size. If you don't see them, you will most likely hear their little peeps and squeaks.

Big Valley is to the right ending in giant granite cliffs. You will hit a long traverse heading west and up to Flattop Mountain. Eventually the trail comes over a ridge and you can actually see Flattop Mountain, although it's not a distinct peak but rather just the flat top stretching out in front of you. The hike steepens for the last mile, crossing a rock field up near the top, and then the long plateau of Flattop Mountain is obvious.

Those wanting to continue can go up another 0.6 miles to the summit of the distinct peak to the left: Hallett Peak. For information on where this trail connects and how to get all the way to the Grand Lake side, refer to my write-up on the overnight hike, Green Mountain Trailhead: Tonahutu Creek Trail to Renegade Campsite to Flattop Mountain (page 157). Otherwise, take a quick rest (to avoid any dangers above tree line: lightning, poor visibility, and more), turn around, and go back down to Bear Lake the way that you came.

DIRECTIONS: From Estes Park go to Rocky Mountain National Park's Beaver Meadows Entrance Station via US 36. After entering the park, go 0.2 miles, take a left at Bear Lake Road, and travel 9.3 miles to the Bear Lake Trailhead parking lot.

GPS Trailhead Coordinates	07 BEAR LAKE TRAILHEAD: FLATTOP MOUNTAIN
UTM zone (WGS84):	13T
Easting:	0445158
Northing:	4462391

o8 Bear Lake Trailhead: *The Loch*

SCENERY: ☆ ☆ ☆ ☆ ☆	DISTANCE: *5.4 miles out–and–back*
TRAIL CONDITION: ☆ ☆ ☆ ☆	HIKING TIME: *3 hours*
CHILDREN: ☆ ☆ ☆	OUTSTANDING FEATURES: *Waterfalls, alpine*
DIFFICULTY: ☆ ☆ ☆	*lake, views*
SOLITUDE: ☆ ☆ ☆	

The Loch is a beautiful mountain lake that's easy to access and popular to photograph. The scenic trail takes hikers past Alberta Falls and away from the Bear Lake and Glacier Gorge Trailhead crowds. The trail can get very warm, so this is a good hike to do when it is overcast or a little bit cool.

🏃 From the Bear Lake Trailhead, cross the wooden bridge and take a left turn. The trail is paved and heads downhill. After about 100 yards, take another left and the trail gradually turns to dirt, but it is so well maintained that you never really notice the difference. After a while, Bear Lake Road is visible on the left, across the river.

Bear right uphill as the trails intersect and follow the signs to Alberta Falls. Stop at the overlook of Alberta Falls or continue to follow the trail uphill to get better views. Social paths lead down to the left to views of various cascades as the trail follows the creek. Stay on the main trail, traveling uphill and then stand above the falls. Hikers are treated to more cascades tumbling down to the left. Alberta Falls are gorgeous and some of the most accessible in Rocky Mountain National Park. Jeweled waters and a narrow gorge make Alberta Falls a classic. Eventually the trail moves away from Glacier Creek, and the views open up to the Mummy Range.

At the next trail junction, bear right and go uphill, following the signs to Mill's Lake and Loch Vale. The cliffs of Glacier Knob are to the right. The trail begins to traverse an old rockslide, which is fairly exposed, but travels back into the shade of the trees. At the

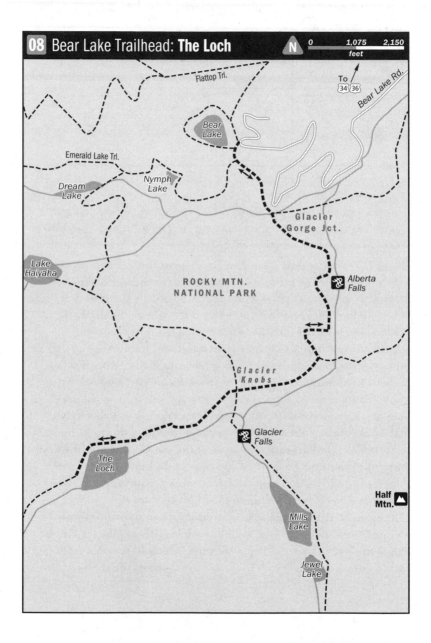

N

0   1,075   2,150
feet

Flattop Trl.

To
34 36

Bear Lake Rd.

Bear
Lake

Emerald Lake Trl.

Dream
Lake

Nymph
Lake

Glacier
Gorge Jct.

Lake
Haiyaha

ROCKY MTN.
NATIONAL PARK

Alberta
Falls

Glacier
Knobs

Glacier
Falls

The
Loch

Half
Mtn.

Mills
Lake

Jewel
Lake

intersection with North Longs Peak Trail, follow the signs to The Loch and Andrews Glacier. The trail is smooth and level, passing in and out of the pine forest.

The trail drops into a subalpine bowl; here Loch Vale and Glacier Gorge come together. A turn to the right takes hikers to Lake Haiyaha and the trail to the left leads into Glacier Gorge. We stay on the middle trail that leads uphill into Loch Vale.

Take the ascending switchbacks above Icy Brook and arrive at The Loch. The Loch is an alpine lake, with crystal clear water, surrounded by snow and views on all sides with Taylor Peak taking center stage. The broad cliff at The Loch is Cathedral Wall, a favorite for technical rock climbers. To the right are Andrews Glacier and Otis Peak. Stop at the piece of land that jets out from the Loch's edge, rest, have lunch, and turn back the way that you came. This area is a good jumping off point to those wanting to continue on to Timberline Falls, Lake of Glass, Sky Pond, and Andrews Glacier. A popular backcountry campsite, Andrews Creek, is 0.6 miles farther up the trail from The Loch.

DIRECTIONS: From Estes Park go to Rocky Mountain National Park's Beaver Meadows Entrance Station via US 36. After entering the park, go 0.2 miles, take a left at Bear Lake Road, and travel 9.3 miles to the Bear Lake Trailhead parking lot.

GPS Trailhead Coordinates	08 BEAR LAKE TRAILHEAD: THE LOCH
UTM zone (WGS84):	13T
Easting:	0445158
Northing:	4462391

SCENERY: ✿ ✿ ✿ ✿	DISTANCE: *4.6 miles out-and-back*
TRAIL CONDITION: ✿ ✿ ✿ ✿	HIKING TIME: *2.5 hours*
CHILDREN: ✿ ✿ ✿ ✿	OUTSTANDING FEATURES: *Moraine Park,*
DIFFICULTY: ✿ ✿	*wildlife, wildflowers, birds, alpine lake*
SOLITUDE: ✿ ✿	

This is an over-the-river-and-through-the-woods hike with a meadow and some elk thrown in. Kids will love this hike, as will those new to hiking and those old to hiking that want to slow down and appreciate the view. Cub Lake is a popular hike, so I recommend that you hike during the week on the shoulder seasons.

🏃🏃 Leave the trailhead and cross the bridge. Pass the sign for Cub Lake that says your destination is reached in 2.4 miles. (The Pool is 3.5 miles; Mill Creek Basin is 4 miles away). The path is double-track and sandy. There is enough room for hikers to walk side by side. Cross another bridge that passes over the Big Thompson River. To the left is the grass and wildflower-filled meadow of the Moraine Park valley. To the immediate right is a forest full of pine trees. Views of Stones Peak, Sprague Mountain, and Gabletop Mountain can been seen from the bridge.

The trail travels up and down at a steady pace, but continues alongside the meadow of Moraine Park. You are not parted from the meadow views until the path goes around a large boulder on man-made stairs, making a sharp turn, thus interrupting the level journey across Moraine Park. Hikers soon travel away from Moraine Park and join up with Cub Creek, heading west.

At the first fork in the trail, take a right turn toward Cub Lake. The trail is now single-track, soft, sandy and travels at a mild ascent. Hike toward the mountains and continue west past the wetlands area.

N

0   800   1,600
feet

To 34 36

P

Fern Lake Rd.

Big Thompson River

Cub Lake Trl.

ROCKY MOUNTAIN
NATIONAL PARK

Cub Lake
Campsite

Cub
Lake

Here you will likely see plenty of ducks in the summer. Elk are notorious for populating this area, especially Moraine Park, all year.

At times, light scrambling over rocks is required. The trail continues to be narrow, rocky, but pretty level. March onward. The path is shaded with a lot of ferns and foliage that hug the side of the trail. We were cruising by on a summer weekday when we came across a couple from Boulder, originally from Germany. He saw our rush and said something profound: "When you stop and sit a minute, you really see things."

The trail begins to ascend through aspen trees and rock piles. As you begin to see more flora and fauna, the trail becomes rockier and little streams pepper the sides. Once we decided to slow down a bit, we did see more. One such find was a number of mountain chickadees we saw peeping around the trail. A single chickadee popped its head in and out of a nest inside the hole of an aspen tree.

The trail switches back two or three times and begins to get steep. (My hiking partner called it an "abrupt change of personality.") Pass the intersection of Cub Lake Trail with the Cub Creek Campsite. Continue straight. Pass another sign pointing to the

Cub Creek Privy. The final destination is Cub Lake. As the name implies, it's a cute little place—not too imposing, but substantial in its own right—with big lily pads, marshy shores, and surrounded on all sides by grass and pine trees. Mountain peaks in view are Stones Peak and Sprague Mountain.

The wildlife at the lake is quite tame, so beware of the ducks and chipmunks when you bring out your food. When we stopped, we were attacked by a ravenous duck.

DIRECTIONS: From Rocky Mountain National Park's Beaver Meadows Entrance, take Bear Lake Road south for 1.2 miles, then turn right toward the Moraine Park Campground. After 0.7 miles, turn left and follow the signs to Cub Lake.

GPS Trailhead Coordinates	09 CUB LAKE TRAILHEAD: CUB LAKE
UTM zone (WGS84):	3T
Easting:	0448060
Northing:	4467390

Deer Mountain

SCENERY: ✧ ✧ ✧ ✧	DISTANCE: *6 miles out-and-back*
TRAIL CONDITION: ✧ ✧ ✧ ✧	HIKING TIME: *3.5 hours*
CHILDREN: ✧ ✧	OUTSTANDING FEATURES: *Meadows, aspen*
DIFFICULTY: ✧ ✧ ✧ ✧	*groves, summit views: Ypsilon Mountain, Longs*
SOLITUDE: ✧ ✧ ✧	*Peak, Estes Park.*

Deer Mountain is a good hike for those wanting a short lung buster with great rewards—the views! Use this hike as a conditioning hike or as a first summit hike for newbies. An early start on a weekday will help avoid the crowds, horses, heat, and afternoon summer thunderstorms.

🚶 Leave the trailhead and head through the scattered ponderosa pine trees and rock outcroppings. The trail is sandy and there is very little foliage surrounding the edges of the trail. Along with the spaciousness at the beginning of the trail comes exposure to the sun. The sun blazes on this first mile, so be sure to have plenty of water. Look to the northwest for the first views of Ypsilon Mountain. Its Y-shaped peak on the face makes it easy to recognize.

At the intersection of Aspen Glen Campground and Deer Mountain Summit take a right, heading toward Deer Mountain. Before the 1-mile point, look downhill toward Beaver Meadows and the views of Longs Peak in the background. A gorgeous aspen grove marches up and down the hill, rounding out a perfect scene.

The forest now offers a short respite in the form of shade. A single switchback changes those plans and sends hikers back across the exposed slope, along the mountainside, traveling at a steep sideways angle as it traverses. The shade reappears, as does a small descent. Don't get too excited because this is your life for the next

N

0   725   1,450
feet

Deer
Mtn.

ROCKY MTN.
NATIONAL PARK

36

34

P

few hours. Up and down, shade and no shade, switchback after switchback—the roller coaster of a summit hike.

The trail levels out 1 mile before the top and tempts hikers with false summits and confusing, sandy side trails. Stay on the main trail (it too is sandy at this point), and continue onward until you reach a sign that marks the right-hand turn to the summit of Deer Mountain. This 0.2 miles path is well earned and a relief, as the summit appears quickly after a short march up a stone stairway.

The Deer Mountain summit is characterized by flat-topped boulders, snaggled trees, and views in all directions. At nearly 10,000 feet, hikers will either be greeted by sunshine and peace or wicked weather complete with whipping winds and lightning strikes. Plan accordingly, because it's always a gamble which one you will get, and that could change in 10 minutes or less. Rest here and turn around, heading the way that you came.

DIRECTIONS: From Rocky Mountain National Park's Beaver Meadows Entrance, take US 36 west to the intersection of US 36 and US 34. Deer Ridge Junction is on the right, before the roads meet. Park in the pull-offs along the shoulder.

GPS Trailhead Coordinates	10 DEER RIDGE JUNCTION TRAILHEAD: DEER MOUNTAIN
UTM zone (WGS84):	13T
Easting:	0448253
Northing:	4470683

East Portal Trailhead: *Wind River and*

Glacier Basin Loop

SCENERY: ☆ ☆ ☆	DISTANCE: *5.06 miles, loop*
TRAIL CONDITION: ☆ ☆ ☆ ☆	HIKING TIME: *2.5 hours*
CHILDREN: ☆ ☆ ☆	OUTSTANDING FEATURES: *River*
DIFFICULTY: ☆ ☆ ☆	
SOLITUDE: ☆ ☆ ☆	

The East Portal Trailhead is run by Larimer County Parks and Recreation and is a nice little park secret. From here, you can access Glacier Basin, the Glacier Creek Trail, the Storm Pass Trail, the Wind River Trail, Emerald Mountain, and two unofficial summits. The loop featured here is a great hike to do if you want to be close to the town of Estes Park, but away from the crowds.

🏃 The trailhead is part of the Alva B. Adams Tunnel property. Part of the Colorado–Big Thompson project, it's one of the main tunnels bringing water from Lake Granby and Shadow Mountain Lake on the west side to the Front Range and the plains. Water exits here, goes down the Big Thompson River to Estes Park and through several power plants all the way down to the lower elevations. The tunnel is 13.1 miles long.

Proceed from the little parking area, which holds about ten cars, on Wind River Trail and cross a small open area with signs notifying you that you are on U.S. Government property but not in Rocky Mountain National Park. The Department of Reclamation maintains the tunnels and owns the land, so the trail signs are not as friendly as those in Rocky Mountain National Park. This trail is also not as well marked as those in Rocky Mountain National Park.

A steady incline brings hikers through sage brush, scattered ponderosa pines, and junipers. Minutes into the hike, pass a sign

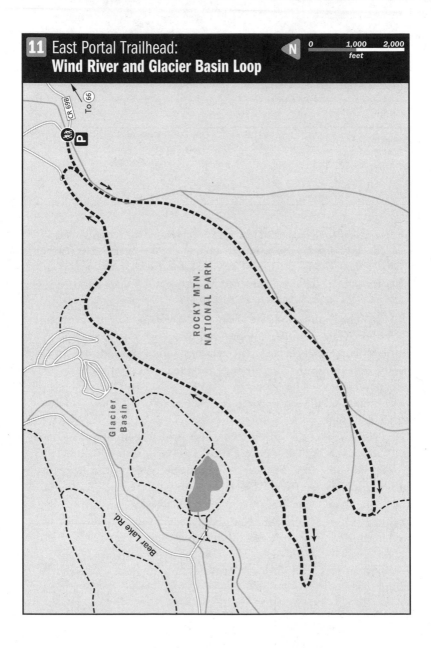

11 East Portal Trailhead:
Wind River and Glacier Basin Loop

N

0   1,000   2,000
feet

CR 69B

To 66

ROCKY MTN.
NATIONAL PARK

Glacier
Basin

Bear Lake Rd.

that says ENTERING ROCKY MOUNTAIN NATIONAL PARK. Continue up about another 100 yards on a sandy and rocky ascent. Come to an intersection where a right turn will take you to the YMCA, and a left, up the hill, goes to Glacier Basin Campground. Take a hard left and traverse the slope, staying on the Wind River Trail.

The trail continues to wind and meander, going a little bit up and then a little bit down. It gets very rocky and goes through some boulders. Another intersection is a trail back down to East Portal Trailhead. Stay on Wind River Trail, veering right on a slight ascent. Hikers enter a more shaded forest here and get out of the sun a little bit. The Wind River cascades off the boulder to the left. Pass a horse hitching rail where there is a single, small campsite, Wind River Bluff, right along the Wind River. Pass two more campsites: Over the Hill and Upper Wind River Site 1. The trail continues a steady ascent. Views of the ridges above open up, and on your left, pass Wind River Site 2. Pass a large and very old aspen grove.

The next intersection is with Storm Pass Trail which leads to Estes Cone. Hikers take a hard right and proceed uphill. Although still wooded, the trail is more exposed to the weather as evidenced by

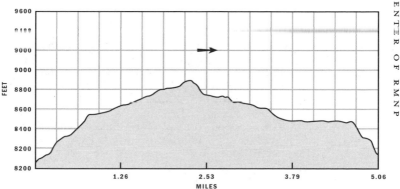

the gnarled trees. Once the trail levels off, keep an eye out for any easy-to-miss right hand turn onto Glacier Basin Trail. Take a hard right here, heading toward the Glacier Basin Campground.

This part of the trail is one of the official cross-country-skiing routes in Rocky Mountain National Park and has orange blaze tags on some of the trees for route finding in the winter. Relatively easy hiking, this part of the trail is more used, especially from people accessing from Bear Lake Road. Continue straight as you pass an intersection with the trail to the left heading over toward Sprague Lake and the more popular trails near Bear Lake Road. Pass another intersection, where a left turn will also take you back toward the Bear Lake Road trails.

You will see a road to your left; it's a park-service campground and maintenance road. Pass a huge metal water tank. Take a right at the intersection with the YMCA Trail, and go uphill. This is a trail used mainly used by the YMCA for its horses. You'll have views of the perfectly conical mountain that is Estes Cone. A quick descent through an aspen grove will take hikers across an open sagebrush-covered slope. Resist the temptation to take a shortcut downhill and go another quarter mile back to the trailhead.

DIRECTIONS: From Estes Park, take US 36 toward Rocky Mountain National Park. Take the first left after Marys Lake Road onto CO 66. Follow the signs to the YMCA. This road becomes County Road 69B. Pass the YMCA and go another mile until the road ends. There is a small day use parking area about 100 yards before the road ends; park here.

GPS Trailhead Coordinates	II EAST PORTAL TRAILHEAD: WIND RIVER AND GLACIER BASIN LOOP
UTM zone (WGS84):	13T
Easting:	450890
Northing:	4464090

Old Forest Inn Campsite

SCENERY: ✿ ✿ ✿ ✿ ✿	DISTANCE: *7.6 miles (2.89 miles to campsite)*
TRAIL CONDITION: ✿ ✿ ✿ ✿	HIKING TIME: *4.5 hours (1.5 hours to campsite)*
CHILDREN: ✿ ✿	OUTSTANDING FEATURES: *Two waterfalls,*
(TO CAMPSITE ✿ ✿ ✿ ✿)	*alpine lake, The Pool, Arch Rocks, Big Thompson*
DIFFICULTY: ✿ ✿ ✿ ✿	*River, Old Forest Inn history*
(TO CAMPSITE ✿ ✿)	
SOLITUDE: ✿ ✿ ✿	

The Old Forest Inn Campsite is the best backcountry site for first-time campers. It's in proximity to Bear Lake access, without the Bear Lake crowds. The beauty of the campsites here attest to the perfect location of an old inn that no longer exists. This hike also offers plenty of easy, yet scenic miles and even more miles of leg-burning uphill. The ascents are rewarded, of course, with the amazing water shows of Marguerite Falls and Fern Falls, and Fern Lake itself. Take the whole family on this outing, camp, split up according to fitness level, and get exploring.

🚶🚶 Leave the trailhead and travel through a forest canopy of various aspen and pine trees. The trail is level for the first mile and very damp, which is uncharacteristic of the Rocky Mountain region. A wide variety of wet, moisture-rich plants live along the banks of the nearby Big Thompson River. Along with the pine and aspen trees, there is a huge variety of trees such as mountain maple trees and river birch trees. Then there are the ferns that carpet the forest ground, thus giving the hike, lake, and falls their namesake.

The trail is single-track packed dirt. Pass by the river on the left and then pass through an old rockslide. The trail is still level, and any type of incline hikers encounter early on is aided by man-made, rock staircases.

12 Fern Lake Trailhead:
Fern Lake and Old Forest Inn Campsite

N

0   1,850   2,700
feet

To 34 36

Fern Lake Rd.

P

Cub Lake Trl.

Cub Lake Campground

Big Thompson River

Cub Lake

Arch Rocks

The Pool

ROCKY MTN. NATIONAL PARK

Old Forest Inn & Campground

Fern Falls

Marguerite Falls

Fern Lake

Continue through a giant boulder field where you wonder, "How did they get here?" These rock formations are so out of place, that the only answer has to be "they got here from outer space." All joking aside, these boulders are part of the Arch Rocks and, according to the park, were part of the early formation of the park, when glaciers melted and big rocks fell to the ground. The giant boulders tower almost 30 feet above hikers, are red in color, and tilt here and there, creating archlike bridges above. There is also a backcountry campsite in this vicinity.

The trail travels along a ridge after Arch Rocks with the Big Thompson River flowing down below. Go straight along a ridge for a while with the river down below.

Pass through another old rockslide and various social trails, staying on the main trail. Come to a large wooden bridge that crosses the Big Thompson River and, more importantly, signifies The Pool. This is a popular destination for school groups and other hikers since it's only 1.5 miles from the trailhead. The Pool is part of an expansive cascade on the river, bordered by a short rock cliff. It's best to stay on the main trail and look at the deep water from the safety of the bridge.

I have never hiked up here and not seen hikers splashing in the water or sliding on embankments or hillsides. One false step and you have a recipe for disaster. Not to mention the impact on the environment.

Cross the bridge at The Pool and take a sharp right turn toward Fern Lake. Head up into the rocks where you will see a sign that says FERN ODESSA. (Fern Lake and Odessa Lake are both lake destinations on this trail.) Cross over the bridge and then arrive at the turn for the Old Forest Inn Campsite.

Overnight Option: Take a right turn and follow the red arrowheads on the trees. There are two sites. The site to the left, or the north, is our favorite because it's representative of the views travelers would have had at the Old Forest Inn. It also has an amazing view of the Big Thompson River below, a gentle river sound, and flat boulders good for camp housekeeping. There are a maximum of two tents at the north site. Higher up on the hill, to the right after turning off the trail, is another campsite that sits above The Pool. This site is a little more exposed, but both sites are in a stand of spruce and fir trees. What is attractive about these sites is that they are easy to get to, but once you get off the trail and up the hill a little bit, all the people disappear.

The Forest Inn was a summer hotel and resort that operated in one form or another until 1949. According to the *Estes Park Trail Gazette*, the buildings were torn down in the spring of 1959 and a calendar found at the site before the demolition was dated 1952. It's interesting to note that there are many lost lodges in Rocky Mountain National Park, including Fern Lodge at Fern Lake, your end hiking destination. Most of these lost lodges were purchased and removed by the park, albeit with much controversy.

Back on Track: After setting up camp or spending the night, the more experienced of your group will continue to Fern Lake. It should be stressed that the ease of the first portion of the trail is by no means representative of the trek to Fern Lake. Let the little ones and the tired ones play, explore, or make lunch around the campsite.

The trail is level and travels along small falls and crosses a split-log bridge. To the left is Fern Falls, and then the real climbing begins. As you approach her, you can hear the sounds of Marguerite Falls. This magnificent water show is worth the effort and a good place to stop and rest. Take the large switchback up the hill after the falls and continue to climb. There is no respite until you get to where the trail intersects with the turn for Spruce Lake and the backcountry campsites for Fern Lake. Continue over the hill to Fern Lake. An old patrol cabin sits to the right. Once you reach the alpine shore of Fern Lake you see Notchtop Mountain and Little Matterhorn rising above the other side of the lake.

After a rest, go back the way you came—downhill this time—to your campsite or the trailhead.

While you are going back, be sure to encourage all the hikers that will undoubtedly ask you "How much farther!?" (The mileage from Fern Falls to Fern Lake is 1 mile. However, the ascent makes it feel farther because hikers are traveling at less than 1.5 miles per hour.)

DIRECTIONS: From the Beaver Meadows Entrance, take Bear Lake Road south for 1.2 miles, and turn right toward Moraine Park Campground. After 0.7 miles, turn left and follow the signs to Cub Lake and Fern Lake. Continue to the Fern Lake Trailhead road and take a left. Travel to the very end of this road and park at the trailhead, an obvious dead end. In the winter, this 0.7-mile stretch is usually closed, so you will have to park at the turnoff where you see the restrooms and a large parking area.

GPS Trailhead Coordinates	12 FERN LAKE TRAILHEAD: FERN LAKE AND OLD FOREST INN CAMPSITE
UTM zone (WGS84):	13T
Easting:	0445770
Northing:	4466970

13 Hollowell Park Trailhead:

Mill Creek Balloon

SCENERY: ✿ ✿ ✿ ✿
TRAIL CONDITION: ✿ ✿ ✿
CHILDREN: ✿ ✿ ✿ ✿
DIFFICULTY: ✿ ✿
SOLITUDE: ✿ ✿ ✿

DISTANCE: *3.4 miles out-and-back*
HIKING TIME: *1.75 hours*
OUTSTANDING FEATURES: *Meadow, aspen trees, views, loop hike, stream, beaver dams*

Loop hikes in Rocky Mountain National Park are rare, so this small balloon hike is a nice change of pace. The fall colors along the Mill Creek Basin are striking because of the patches of aspens that make their home here. Novice hikers will appreciate the scenery and the ease of this trail. Seasoned hikers like this trail for its access to other areas of the park, its beauty, and the surprising lack of crowds even with the proximity to the park entrance.

🚶🚶 Leave the trailhead and enter into the meadow where dry grasses are framed by views of the surrounding moraines. The trail is sandy and dusty, yet smooth and level. If there is no rain, hikers will kick up a lot of dust onto their hiking boots in this section.

Look for the strip of aspen trees on Bierstadt Moraine that is especially striking in September, when the aspen leaves turn golden. The light-colored trees growing on the forest's slope are aspens that mark an old logging skid trial. Lumbermen hauled timbers from the saw mill up near Bierstadt Lake to build the Stanley Hotel.

The trail is still on level ground as it continues to pass through the silver and green sagebrush that lines the path. Pine trees begin to close in on the openness of the trail, although it still offers views of Longs Peak to the left. Continue straight at the intersection of Hollowell Park Trail, Mill Creek Basin, and the horse trail to Moraine Park, which makes a sharp right behind you.

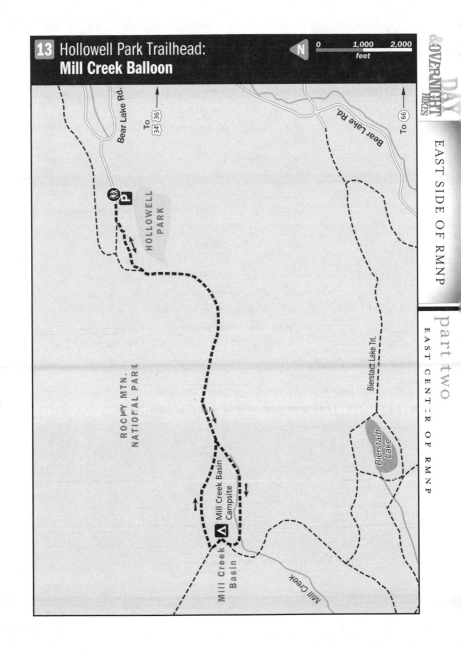

13 Hollowell Park Trailhead: Mill Creek Balloon

N

0   1,000   2,000
feet

EAST SIDE OF RMNP

part two
EAST CENTER OF RMNP

Bear Lake Rd.

To 34 36

Bear Lake Rd.

To 66

HOLLOWELL PARK

ROCKY MTN. NATIONAL PARK

Bierstadt Lake Trl.

Bierstadt Lake

Mill Creek Basin Campsite

Mill Creek Basin

Mill Creek

Once the trail gets closer to Mill Creek, social trails travel away from the main trail. Stay on the main trail as it begins to make a gradual climb through the trees.

At the intersection of Mill Creek Basin, Bierstadt Lake, Bear Lake, Cub Lake, and Hollowell Park, take a left turn across the bridge and continue on. The trail to the right is where you will come down completing the balloon portion of the loop. (If you prefer an intense elevation gain and a more difficult hike, take a right turn here and travel counterclockwise around the balloon.)

The trail travels at a slight ascent and is full of rocks. The erosion here is a telltale sign that there is a lot of runoff in this area when the rainwater comes through. Hikers step over a lot of stuff in this section including rocks and tree roots. The trail rolls on, gets sandy and flat for a spell, and then continues to travel upward.

Take a right turn heading toward Mill Creek Basin Campsite and Cub Lake at the next junction where Hollowell Park, Bear Lake, Bierstadt Lake, Upper Mill Creek, Cub Lake, and Mill Creek Basin all intersect. This marks the 1.7-mile point. Mill Creek Basin is a meadow framed by Mount Wuh to the west and Steep Mountain to

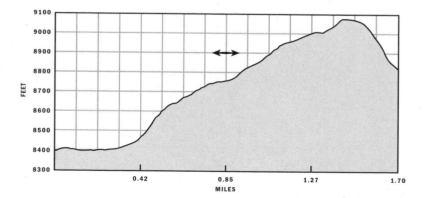

the northeast. When you get to the next intersection, take a right turn and head in a clockwise pattern back to the main trail. Cross over the creek via a bridge and pass a horse hitch on the right.

The trail travels through short meadows and trees now. Take a sharp right and continue to Hollowell Park at the intersection of Hollowell Park, Cub Lake, and Mill Creek Basin Campsite. The trail ascends one more time, levels out, and drops us back down to where we came from. The trail descends sharply, is very steep, and not in the best condition. What is striking is how the aspen trees frame the trail—they look like they are standing in wait as you head downward. The aspen trees through here are uncharacteristically big and old. Eventually you reach the forest floor and get to walk alongside the trees. Then you will meet up with the main trail where you head straight back to the trailhead by retracing your steps.

DIRECTIONS: From the Beaver Meadows Entrance, take Bear Lake Road south for 3.5 miles. Turn right at the Hollowell Park Trailhead. Drive a few hundred yards to the parking area.

GPS Trailhead Coordinates	TO HOLLOWELL PARK
	TRAILHEAD: MILL CREEK
	BALLOON
UTM zone (WGS84):	13T
Easting:	0448650
Northing:	4465632

Ute Meadows Loop

SCENERY: ✵ ✵ ✵ ✵	DISTANCE: *8.5 miles out-and-back*
TRAIL CONDITION: ✵ ✵ ✵	HIKING TIME: *5 hours*
CHILDREN: ✵ ✵	OUTSTANDING FEATURES: *Meadow,*
DIFFICULTY: ✵ ✵ ✵ ✵	*forest, wildlife, stream, views of Longs Peak and*
SOLITUDE: ✵ ✵ ✵	*Deer Mountain*

The Upper Beaver Meadows loop is a nice hike in its own right, but when you add the spur to the Ute Meadows Campsite it makes it that much more interesting. The Beaver Meadows portion is mostly arid, with sweeping views of the heart of Rocky Mountain National Park. The trek to the Ute Meadows Campsite is an uphill hike and quite a challenge with backpacking gear. The campsite is llama accessible, so this may be your chance to have someone, or something else, pack it in.

🚶🚶 Leave the trailhead and follow the signs to the Ute Meadows Campsite, staying on the right-hand trail when the path makes its immediate split. This is the intersection of Beaver Meadows Trailhead, Moraine Park, Ute Meadows Campsite, and Trail Ridge Road. The trails seem to meander in and out at this point, so it is important to remember to stay in a direction that heads toward the Ute Trail.

The trail is wide and sandy at the beginning. It then begins to turn into a single-track, ascending at a gentle grade as the views of Moraine Valley to the left gradually begin to disappear. Start to travel through the forest. After 1.5 miles, reach the junction of Beaver Meadows Trailhead, Ute Meadows Campsite, and Trail Ridge Road. It is now another 1.2 miles to the campsite. Take the left trail heading forward on the Ute Trail.

The views to the left now open up to Longs Peak and Mount Meeker as the path enters the Windy Gulch area. The trail has a very

14 Upper Beaver Meadows Trailhead:
Ute Meadows Loop

N

0   0.3   0.6
feet

Deer Mtn.

36

Beaver Meadows

To 34

Fern Lake Rd.

P

Beaver Meadows Trailhead

ROCKY MTN. NATIONAL PARK

Beaver Mtn.

Ute Meadows Campsite

steep ascent right after the intersection. Don't forget to look out at the views as you catch your breath. As you gain elevation, the views below are of the Cub Lake area. The path is faint and hard to follow in spots.

The trail then opens up, looking west to the timberline area of Trail Ridge. The path begins to travel over rocks, and hikers may be required to scramble over a few. Keep an eye out for cairns as a tool for staying on track while in the rocks. The trail then makes a quick descent and travels along a small stream that is very shaded. The next intersection is an indicator for Beaver Mountain Trailhead, 2.8 miles (this is how far we have come) and Trail Ridge Road, 3.8 miles. This is where you will take a left turn into the campsite.

The Ute Meadows Campsite is a beautiful camping area located in a dry, sandy area. After crossing a small stream to get to the site, the forest will be to the left and the meadow to the right. The trees that dot the right-hand side obscure the views of the meadow. After a night's rest, we will turn back onto the Ute Trail and head back the way that we came. Hikers may be curious as to where the Ute Trail goes if you continue the other direction. The trail travels over

Timberline Pass, through Tombstone Ridge, ending at the Ute
Crossing Trailhead on Trail Ridge Road.

After backtracking, arrive at the junction of the Ute Trail and
Upper Beaver Meadows. Take a left turn to begin a clockwise loop
around Upper Beaver Meadows. The turn says that it is 3.5 miles to
the Upper Beaver Meadows Trailhead. The trail travels at a slow, but
nice ascent and views to the right are of Longs Peak. The trail then
enters the sun; travels through small, forested pockets; and continues
onward.

Cross two streams and then travel down into a meadow where the
trail is sandy. The trail then begins another moderate climb through
the forest. You can now see Trail Ridge Road in some spots and the
first sightings of Deer Mountain. The trail is very exposed, in an
open meadow as you pass the intersection with Deer Ridge Junction.
Stay on the main trail and travel back to the Upper Beaver Meadows
Trailhead in a descent through the meadow. The trail ends on the
access road, and you must walk the last 50 feet on the pavement back
to your car.

DIRECTIONS: From the Beaver Meadows Entrance, take US 36 west
to the turn off for the Upper Beaver Meadows Trailhead, just before
the junction with US 34. Turn left onto the dirt road and take it for
2 miles until it ends at the parking lot and trailhead.

GPS Trailhead Coordinates

14 UPPER BEAVER MEADOWS
TRAILHEAD: UTE MEADOWS
LOOP

UTM zone (WGS84):	13T
Easting:	0447931
Northing:	4469143

3

Southeast Side of Rocky Mountain National Park

Longs Peak Area and Wild Basin Area

More
than 110
mountai
peak
towe
ove
the 415
squar
miles o
hiking
trails
picni
spots
waterfalls
cold lakes
an
bountifu
wildlif

15 Lily Lake Trailhead: *Lily Ridge Trail*

SCENERY: ☆ ☆ ☆ ☆
TRAIL CONDITION: ☆ ☆ ☆ ☆
CHILDREN: ☆ ☆ ☆ ☆ ☆
DIFFICULTY: ☆
SOLITUDE: ☆ ☆

DISTANCE: *1.34 miles, loop*
HIKING TIME: *45 minutes*
OUTSTANDING FEATURES: *Lake, views*

Lily Ridge Trail offers hikers a little variety to the hike around Lily Lake. It gives novice hikers their first experience with an ascent and gets kids out of the stroller and onto the trail. This is a popular spot for anglers, picnickers, and hikers. Anglers line the shore and can be found bobbing around in individual fishing tubes.

The trailhead and parking area for Lily Lake are across the road from Lily Lake Visitor Center, which is currently closed. Leave the trailhead; turn right onto the trail directly along the perimeter of the lake. Take a right turn before the wooden bridge at the sign that says LILY RIDGE TRAIL. Start heading upward at a gradual ascent. Continue on gentle switchbacks and scramble over the rock steps in the path.

The Lily Ridge Trail travels from the east end of Lily Lake to its west end along the ridge to the north of the lake. Immediately look out across Lily Lake toward Longs Peak. Begin to head away from the views of the lake and up over a fake summit and ridge. Now you will glance toward Estes Park and see the rooftops of Camp Cheley.

The trail levels off and heads west along the ridge a few hundred feet above the lake. Cross up through large rocks to a small bench that offers a nice respite and fantastic views of Longs Peak. Continue along the counterclockwise loop on the ridge along the trail.

Descent begins around the backside of the lake, on the west end. The descent is gradual and easy on the legs. Hikers now start back for the shores of Lily Lake. This lake is the beginning of Fish Creek

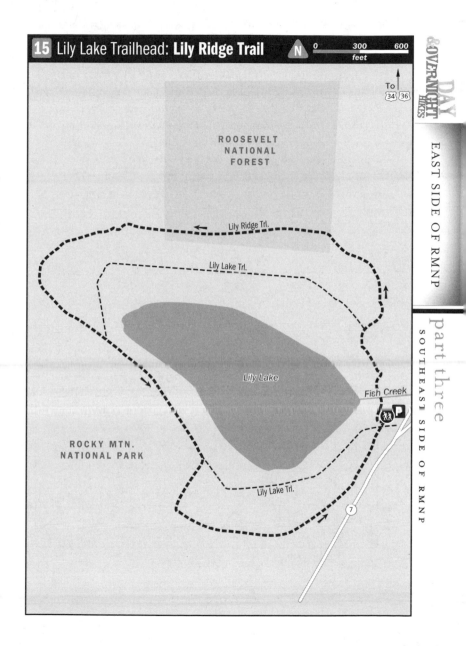

To
34 36

ROOSEVELT
NATIONAL
FOREST

Lily Ridge Trl.

Lily Lake Trl.

Lily Lake

Fish Creek

Lily Lake Trl.

ROCKY MTN.
NATIONAL PARK

7

which flows into Lake Estes. The Lily Lake Trail is wheelchair accessible, wide, level, and lined by logs.

Pass the intersection of Lily Ridge Trail and Lily Lake Trail. You'll want to continue straight and then make a left turn to stay on the Lily Lake Trail. The Lily Ridge Trail is complete at this point. Do not go right onto the service road. From this vantage point you can see the Twin Sisters Peaks toward the east.

At the next trail intersection take the right-hand spur that heads south to more shade and nice picnic spots with tables. Keep following this trail until you return back to the parking area and trailhead.

DIRECTIONS: From Estes Park, go south on CO 7, past Marys Lake. The road curves sharply and travels to Lily Lake Visitor Center on the left. Turn right here and park in the small lot across the street and adjacent to the lake.

GPS Trailhead Coordinates	15 LILY LAKE TRAILHEAD:
	LILY RIDGE TRAIL
UTM zone (WGS84):	13T
Easting:	454346
Northing:	4461734

16 Lily Lake Trailhead : *Twin Sisters Peaks*

SCENERY: ☆ ☆ ☆
TRAIL CONDITION: ☆ ☆ ☆
CHILDREN: ☆
DIFFICULTY: ☆ ☆ ☆ ☆
SOLITUDE: ☆ ☆

DISTANCE: *8 miles out-and-back*
HIKING TIME: *4 hours*
OUTSTANDING FEATURES: *Views of Estes Park, Rocky Mountain National Park; optimal views of Longs Peak; mostly shaded*

The Twin Sisters sit at the easternmost edge of Rocky Mountain National Park and are accessed without entering the park. The trail winds through forest with some of the best panoramic views of Longs Peak. This is a great conditioning climb for those wanting to tackle considerable elevations.

Start at Lily Lake Visitor Center. The former Twin Sisters Trail, which began directly west of the summit in Tahosa Valley, has been abandoned by the National Park Service. Park at the Lily Lake Visitor Center and hike the extra 0.3 miles to avoid the nightmare parking along the road, right before the true trailhead. Get on the road right behind the visitor center and follow it away from the highway. At the official trailhead for Twin Sisters, take a left onto the trail. Start out on a small service road bordered on both sides by a new evergreen tree growth. Immediately on the left is a small wooden bridge, Twin Sisters Trail information, and a trail marker.

Start a steady ascent on a trail comprised of loose rock and dirt. Enter a pine forest and then enter Forest Service land as the trees crowd and condense around the trail. Hikers ascend rather quickly and must scramble across some early rocks. The trail takes a deep right switchback and continues up the face of the mountain. The ascending path is aided in spots, not only by switchbacks, but also by man-placed rock staircases. Continue to climb as scenery stays the same. Cross a rock slide and enter into Rocky Mountain National Park. The trail becomes much steeper here, with a large staircase looming in the distance.

16 Lily Lake Trailhead: **Twin Sisters Peaks** N

0   950   1,900
feet

To 34 36

S. Saint Vrain Ave.

Fish Creek Rd.

Lily Lake

Lily Lake
Visitor Center
(closed)

P

ROOSEVELT
NATIONAL FOREST

ROCKY MTN.
NATIONAL PARK

7

Wind River Pass

Lookout
Springs

Old Twin Sisters Trl. (Closed)

Butterfly
Burn

Twin Sisters
Peaks

Turn and look to the right to capture the first amazing views of Longs Peak as it rises up over the Tahosa Valley. Pass through a second rockslide. Reach a small overlook and take in the view. Continue on as the trail starts a gradual descent, which is welcome since the previous steps have been straight uphill.

Pass a huge, five-story-tall boulder and then take artificially carved rock stairs up. The trail switches back again to the left and continues an uphill climb. Aspen trees have now begun to mix in with the tall, dense evergreens. Smaller switchbacks continue, and the trail is very rocky with exposed tree roots.

The trail continues its upward journey and then reaches an area where there are fewer trees, more shrubs, and small aspens. The trail is narrow and hard to navigate due to huge rocks in the path. Climb away from the hillside and leave the view of Longs Peak. Enter Forest Service land again and continue. After passing through the timberline, keep going to the summit area and head past the communications tower. The true Twin Sisters summit is not directly accessible by trail, but can be reached by a brief scramble heading east from the communications tower. Take in the views and head back the way that you came.

DIRECTIONS: From Estes Park, go south on CO 7, past Marys Lake. The road curves sharply and travels to Lily Lake Visitor Center on the left. Turn in here and park.

GPS Trailhead Coordinates	16 LILY LAKE TRAILHEAD: TWIN SISTERS PEAKS
UTM zone (WGS84):	13T
Easting:	454440
Northing:	4461730

SCENERY: ✰ ✰ ✰	DISTANCE: *5 miles out-and-back*
TRAIL CONDITION: ✰ ✰ ✰ ✰	HIKING TIME: *2.5 hours*
CHILDREN: ✰ ✰ ✰	OUTSTANDING FEATURES: *Shaded alpine*
DIFFICULTY: ✰ ✰ ✰	*forest, views of Estes Park and Rocky Mountain*
SOLITUDE: ✰ ✰ ✰ ✰	*National Park*

Lily Mountain is ideal for Estes Park visitors who don't have the time to hike in the heart of Rocky Mountain National Park. This is a classic alpine hike with reward-ing views and a steady climb. Lily Mountain is often passed over for other hikes in the vicinity, such as Twin Sisters, and the hike is often confused with the small walk around Lily Lake. In addition, it's usually kept a secret and out of brochures, making this hike one of the least crowded around Estes Park.

🚶🚶 Leave the parking area and begin to climb directly from the trailhead. (There are no facilities here, only a call box. Parking is also very limited.) Pass a National Park Service boundary post and a Lily Mountain sign. The first half mile parallels CO 7 as the shaded trail begins its ascent along the ridge. Large pines and boulder clusters dominate the landscape here. The hard-packed-dirt trail has loose rocks and some exposed tree roots. Expect snow on the trail if you hike outside of the recommended seasons. We hiked in early winter and encountered packed snow from the trailhead on.

Early in the trail the landscape also includes aspen trees and consistent light filtering through the trees. The trail takes an unchar-acteristic dip and then flattens out before ascending a small man-made staircase and starting a series of small switchbacks. As the trail crests, the Estes Park Valley, Marys Lake, and the southern portion of the town of Estes Park come into view. Pass a natural break in the trail that has been carved by hikers going off of the trail to the right

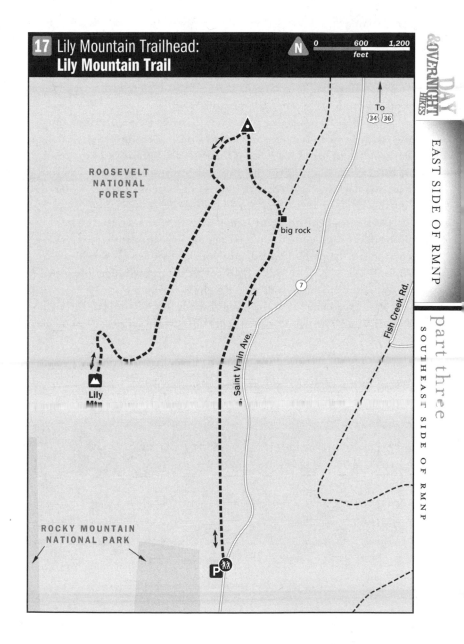

17 Lily Mountain Trailhead:
Lily Mountain Trail

N

0   600   1,200
feet

To
34 36

ROOSEVELT
NATIONAL
FOREST

big rock

7

Fish Creek Rd.

Saint Vrain Ave.

Lily
Mtn

ROCKY MOUNTAIN
NATIONAL PARK

P

and continue to the left. This boulder-shaded spot is a nice place for a rest. From this junction, start another gradual climb toward Lily Mountain. The summit is not yet in view. Continue on the trail and pass more large rocks and a picturesque dead tree that stands as a sentinel on the right after a large switchback.

At a large outcropping of boulders, you'll see an overlook on the right. Look to the left for views of Rocky Mountain National Park and right for more views of the Estes Park Valley and the town of Estes Park. Get back on the trail and continue to climb. The trail becomes dark and shaded, with a forest of large pine trees clustered together.

As the trail continues to ascend with switchbacks, there are built-in erosion-control devices, mainly logs and landscaping materials, along the path. This side of the ridge can be very windy, and you will hear the wind whipping through the dense lodgepole pines. You'll also hear the sounds of the highway far below.

Pass a trail marker at the crest of the hill. Continue to the right toward Lily Mountain's peak, which consists of a large rock pile.

Cairns mark the route to the top and hikers must scramble up this last part of the trail.

Views from the top are extraordinary and include Longs Peak, Twin Sisters, and the Mummy Range. After photographs, maybe lunch, and a rest, turn around to retrace the same route.

DIRECTIONS: From Estes Park, go south on CO 7, past Marys Lake. The road curves sharply. After 4.8 miles, look for a small parking area on the right shoulder of the road and Lily Mountain Trail marker.

GPS Trailhead Coordinates	17 LILY MOUNTAIN TRAILHEAD: LILY MOUNTAIN
UTM zone (WGS84):	13T
Easting:	454560
Northing:	4462470

SCENERY: ☆ ☆ ☆ ☆	DISTANCE: *15 miles out-and-back*
TRAIL CONDITION: ☆ ☆ ☆	HIKING TIME: *12 hours*
CHILDREN: ☆	OUTSTANDING FEATURES: *Fourteener,*
DIFFICULTY: ☆ ☆ ☆ ☆ ☆	*evergreen forest, lakes, spectacular mountain views,*
SOLITUDE: ☆ ☆	*tundra, waterfalls*

The excursion up this awe-inspiring mountain blurs the lines between a hike and a climb. The 15 miles will likely rank among the most spectacular yet hard-earned miles you have ever hiked. This mountain displays both imposing stature and magnificent beauty that validate its popularity. Longs Peak is the tallest mountain in Rocky Mountain National Park and the fourteener that sits farthest north in Colorado. It is also the easternmost point of the Continental Divide.

🏃 Leave the trailhead and follow the East Longs Peak Trail (Keyhole Route) and begin an enchanting jaunt through the trees. Pass a small campground named Goblins Forest. At 1.9 miles, reach a well-constructed bridge crossing over a small cascading waterfall. This is a beautiful place to take a break.

Your first views of Longs Peak are here as the trees transition to shorter vegetation. At 2.5 miles, there is a fork in the trail. Follow the sign left toward the summit. After another mile, you'll reach the junction of the Chasm Lake Trail. This is another great spot to rest, because there is a pit toilet and a vista of the east Diamond face of Longs Peak. Head northwest as the trail skirts up Mount Lady Washington to Granite Pass.

Stay left and hike southwest for 1.7 miles to the boulder field. Within this field are another pit toilet and several rock shelters that act as a windbreak for tents. The boulder field consists of car-sized boulders. Begin to scramble your way straight up toward the Keyhole.

N

0   0.37   0.75
miles

Gillette Dr.

7

To 34/36

Longs Peak Rd.

Longs Peak Ranger Station

P

Storm Pass Trl.

Inn Brook

Eugenia Mine

Pine Ridge

Longs Peak Trl.

Mills Moraine

Roaring Fork

Larimer County

Boulder County

Columbine Falls

Battle Mtn.

Granite Pass

Mt. Lady Washington

Chasm Lake

ROCKY MTN. NATIONAL PARK

Longs Peak

Mt. Meeker

The Narrows

Storm Peak

The Keyhole

The Trough

At the base of the Boulder Field, the top of Longs Peak, the Keyhole, and the expanse of the boulder field are visible.

Many people choose to backpack this far to make for a shorter climb the next day. All campers must obtain a Backcountry Wilderness Use Permit. Be warned that you are camping well above tree line and the surface area is 100 percent rock.

The impressive view of the Longs Peak summit is highlighted here by a rock formation aptly dubbed the Keyhole. At the Keyhole is a small, stone shelter. The terrain becomes significantly more difficult beyond the Keyhole, so take a moment to evaluate the time, the weather, and your physical condition. There is no shame in turning back if the conditions aren't right, so don't let pride get in the way of wisdom.

Cross through the Keyhole to the west side of the ridge and glance at an expansive view of Glacier Gorge. The trail is now marked by bull's-eyes painted on the rocks. The remainder of the trail is extremely slick when wet and very exposed to the elements. A fall here could be fatal. Follow the exposed ledge for just over a quarter mile

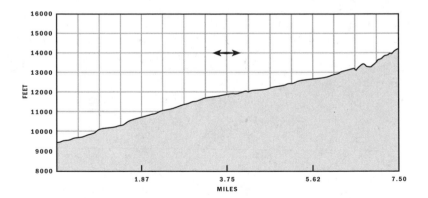

to a large couloir called the Trough. Ascend the Trough to the top of the west ridge.

Now the trail will traverse east across Longs Peak's south face using a ledge called the Narrows. This ledge is narrow—only one hiker wide—and exposed. Take your time and stay calm.

Beyond the Narrows lies the Homestretch. The Homestretch leads you northeast by a series of steep, slick, angled slabs. Be mindful of loose rock; tread lightly, and watch for rock kicked loose by other hikers. In a short time, the summit of Longs Peak seems to just magically appear. This airy pinnacle is large and flat. The commanding panorama is well-deserved compensation for your sweat and tired legs. At 14,255 feet, there are plenty of photo opportunities.

After celebration of your lofty accomplishment, turn around and head back the way you came. The ascent will most likely be crowded, which can be a problem on the narrow ledges where hikers cannot pass each other.

Note: Hiking time and terrain warrant extra consideration when preparing for this outing. A headlamp is useful for an early start, which is essential for a successful completion of this hike. Many hikers begin as early as 2 a.m. Equip yourself with ample layers of clothing and extra food and water; this is a long one. As always, tell someone where you're going and when you expect to be back. An average of 60 search and rescue incidents occur per year on this peak alone. Crowds of hikers fill this trail every day. Be prepared for a lot of human contact. Snow is often found on this hike, especially through the Trough portion, at any time during the hiking season. I recommend hiking Longs Peak in June through October.

Overnight Option: Longs Peak Campground

Go to bed early. The park service recommends that you try to leave the trailhead between 3 a.m. and 6 a.m. to make it to the summit of Longs Peak by noon. Bad weather can occur at any time but is more likely in the afternoon during the summer. Bring plenty of warm clothes and plenty of lung power. The round-trip lasts from 12 to 15 hours. Make sure to keep your campsite a second night because you will be too exhausted to do anything except make supper and hit the sack.

This tents-only camping area is located in a scenic setting adjacent to some of the most beautiful mountain land in the Rockies. There are many sights to see and things to do, but the very things that attract you to this park also attract many other visitors. Longs Peak is an extremely popular hike here. Cars will line the road leading to the trailhead and campground. It takes a combination of timing and luck to get a campsite during the peak season, which is from late June through mid-September. All sites are first come, first served. When you do get a campsite, you will realize that in spite of all the cars nearby, the hustle and bustle won't overwhelm you in this 26-site campground.

The trailhead parking area, however, will have all the hustle and bustle. Pass the line of parked cars along Longs Peak Road and come to a split in the road. Turn right and enter the campground. To your left is the always-full-during-the-summer trailhead parking. The teardrop-shaped gravel campground loop makes its way beneath a lodgepole woodland pocked with boulders and smaller trees. The campsites are mostly on the outside of the loop and have somewhat obstructed views of the Twin Sisters peaks across the Tahosa Valley in the Roosevelt National Forest.

More campsites are stretched along the peak side of the loop. As popular as they are, they are well maintained. A hill rises against the campground. This is the campground's rockier side; campsites are more spread out over here. Overall, the sites are average in size, with ample room for the average tent. But always being full does make the place seem a bit confined. Colorful tents and colorful people give Longs Peak some extra pizzazz.

DIRECTIONS: From Estes Park, go south on CO 7, past Marys Lake. The road curves sharply and travels to the Longs Peak Trailhead turnoff. Turn right here and travel 1 mile to the Longs Peak Trailhead.

GPS Trailhead Coordinates	18 LONGS PEAK TRAILHEAD: LONGS PEAK
UTM zone (WGS84):	13T
Easting:	0452659
Northing:	4457866

Storm Pass to Estes Cone

SCENERY: ✿ ✿ ✿ ✿	DISTANCE: *6.7 miles out-and-back*
TRAIL CONDITION: ✿ ✿ ✿ ✿	HIKING TIME: *3.5 hours*
CHILDREN: ✿ ✿	OUTSTANDING FEATURES: *Shaded evergreen*
DIFFICULTY: ✿ ✿ ✿ ✿	*forest with spectacular mountain views at the top*
SOLITUDE: ✿ ✿ ✿	

Estes Cone is an inactive volcano cone. In this book we will profile the trail from Longs Peak Trailhead, even though there are two other access points to Estes Cone. This mostly shaded trail is a nice hike in the summer. It's also a good hike early or late in the season, when some other nearby hikes are thick with snow or impassable due to snow. Estes Cone is a Rocky Mountain National Park hike that can be accessed here without an entrance fee.

🚶 Follow Longs Peak Trail from behind the little ranger's display and miniature museum at the parking lot. Please stop to sign in at the trail register right by the trailhead. Immediately ascend well-maintained, man-made stairs. Since the trail is in Rocky Mountain National Park, hikers can expect a well-kept path throughout this hike, although the last half mile is rocky, steep, and hard to navigate.

The first half mile of trail is a steady, moderate grade that intersects with Storm Pass Trail. Take a right here onto Storm Pass Trail and follow the signs to Estes Cone.

The trail slowly gives way to loose rock and exposed tree roots. The grade varies as well, including some short descents, and traverses below Pine Ridge. Cross Inn Brook using a log bridge and continue to the right of an abandoned log cabin site with a rusted boiler and tailings. This is all that remains of the Eugenia Mine.

19 Longs Peak Trailhead:
Storm Pass to Estes Cone

N

0   975   1,950
feet

DAY
&OVERNIGHT
HIKES

EAST SIDE OF RMNP

part three

SOUTHEAST SIDE OF RMNP

Estes
Cone

Storm Pass Trl.

Eugenia
Mine

log bridge

Inn Brook

Storm Pass Trl.

ROCKY MTN.
NATIONAL PARK

Storm Pass Trl.

Goblins Castle Rd.

Longs Peak Trl.

Longs Peak
Ranger Station

P

To
7

Longs Peak
Rd.

The trail starts a descent that seems a little out of place, since our goal is to travel to a summit. Continue to drop down and cross a small meadow as the trail opens up to views of Twin Sisters and our destination, Estes Cone. The trail becomes sandy and smooth. Pass the Moore Park campsites and at mile 2 reach a trail spur. Take a left, follow the signs to Estes Cone, and begin a sharp ascent toward Storm Pass. It is from this point that the trail makes up for lost time and gains most of its elevation.

To the left are spectacular views. The mountain to your far left is Mount Meeker. Longs Peak can be spotted poking above the ridge, with the peak's diamond facing the trail.

Lungs begin to tire as the elevation climbs and the trees become visibly shorter and stunted. At 2.5 miles, you reach the pass, marked by large rock cairns and signs. The Storm Pass Cutoff, to the right, is accessed at the Lily Lake Trailhead. Follow the signs to Estes Cone Trail, bearing right up through rock cairns and the stunted evergreens that dot the hillside. Estes Cone is straight ahead, and once out of the trees, the trail begins to ascend the cone's southwest flank.

The trail is steep and rocky, with twisted and stunted wind-worn trees. A close look at some of these trees will show lightning damage.

Continue to follow the cairns as you pick your way through a vertical rock garden for the last half mile. Eventually, reach a small flat area, then head up and right and scramble through rocks to the summit of Estes Cone. You are rewarded with magnificent views of Estes Park, Rocky Mountain National Park, Longs Peak, and Mount Meeker. But you should head down, back to the trailhead, before afternoon lightning storms return as they do most of the summer.

The trailhead has a ranger station with a ranger usually on duty; restrooms; campsites; picnic facilities; and a museum, which has plentiful information on hikes and Rocky Mountain National Park.

This hike shares a trailhead with Longs Peak Trail, a very popular hike. Many people start Longs Peak Trail at 4 or 5 a.m., finishing in early evening. Parking is limited, sometimes freeing up in the afternoon. However, an early start is recommended because lightning storms are common after 12 p.m. The best months to hike here are May through October.

DIRECTIONS: From Estes Park, turn left off US 36 onto CO 7 before the town's first stoplight. Go south on CO 7, past Marys Lake. The road curves sharply and travels to the Longs Peak Trailhead turnoff. Turn right here and travel 1 mile to the Longs Peak Trailhead.

GPS Trailhead Coordinates	19 LONGS PEAK TRAILHEAD: STORM PASS TO ESTES CONE
UTM zone (WGS84):	13T
Easting:	0452659
Northing:	4457866

20 Sandbeach Lake Trailhead:

Sandbeach Lake

SCENERY: ☆ ☆ ☆ ☆	DISTANCE: *9 miles out-and-back*
TRAIL CONDITION: ☆ ☆ ☆	HIKING TIME: *5 hours*
CHILDREN: ☆ ☆ ☆	OUTSTANDING FEATURES: *Unique alpine*
DIFFICULTY: ☆ ☆ ☆	*lake setting, headwaters of Sandbeach Creek, views*
SOLITUDE: ☆ ☆ ☆ ☆	*of North St. Vrain Creek drainage, Campers Creek,*
	Hunters Creek

The sandy shore of Sandbeach Lake is a nice reward for this uphill trek. And that's a good thing, since the elevation gain on this hike is almost 2,000 feet. Its trailhead location, nestled in the south side of Mount Meeker, is a quiet setting for a day hike or an overnight camping trip. The Wild Basin area, near Allenspark, is usually not crowded and is reminiscent of the earlier days in the park. Sandbeach Lake Trail is an easy trail to follow since there are four landmarks that are spaced pretty evenly apart. The first is a trail intersection at 1.5 miles, a creek crossing at 1 more mile, another creek crossing in another mile, and then the lake in 1 more mile.

🏃 Starting from the parking lot, the trail switches back a few times and continues through the forest along Copeland Moraine. Reach a ridgetop after 1.5 miles, pass an intersection with the Meeker Park trails, and take a left. The trail is very rocky and continues to travel along the ridge in this first section. Copeland Lake is visible on the left.

As you climb, and the trail rises steeply from the valley, be sure to look back to the left for views of the North St. Vrain Creek drainage, filled with beaver ponds. To the west are views of Mount Copeland. We hiked in the fall when the colors were turning along the trail and in the entire drainage area. The aspen trees were golden, while the brush along the drainage was already a blaze of orange and red.

20 Sandbeach Lake Trailhead:
Sandbeach Lake

N

0   0.35   0.7
miles

To 34 36

MEEKER PARK

Copeland Dam

CR 115

Horsetooth Peak

Lookout Mtn.

Campers Creek

Wild Basin Ranger Station

ROCKY MTN. NATIONAL PARK

Hunters Creek

Sandbeach Creek

Lyric Falls

Sandbeach Lake

7

Pass the Hole in the Wall Campsite. The trail is now flat and very sandy. Continue west along the Sandbeach Lake Trail as it passes alongside of Lookout Mountain. Rock outcroppings tower above the trail as it travels along a sandy path that leads through a spruce and pine tree forest.

Pass Campers Creek Campsite, almost a mile from the Meeker Park intersection. Travel along the shaded creek, down a sharp descent. Cross the waters of Campers Creek on a footbridge and then go back up the hill on the other side of the creek. Pass Beaver Mill Campsite and Hunters Creek Campsite. You will then cross the actual waters of Hunters Creek; you have traveled a mile since the last creek crossing.

West of Hunters Creek, the trail gets steep and climbs 1 more mile to Sandbeach Lake. You'll know you are close when you pass a horse hitch rack on the right. Arrive at Sandbeach Lake. As its namesake suggests, the shoreline is a large, sandy beach. The views to the north are of Longs Peak, Mount Meeker, Keyboard of the Winds, and Pagoda Mountain. On the west side it is forested, while the east side is home to the aforementioned sandy shore.

Like many high altitude lakes, Sandbeach Lake was dammed in the early 1900s to help provide water to the Colorado Front Range. The lake was filled at one point, but the National Park Service bought the reservoir and took apart the dam in the 1980s. The sandy shore was exposed at that time when the water receded.

After a visit to the shore and a nice rest, turn back around the way that you came and return to the trailhead. There is a group campsite and an individual campsite in nice proximity to Sandbeach Lake. If you'd rather extend your hike and take advantage of the unique setting that Sandbeach Lake offers, then get a backcountry permit and stay awhile. Many also use Sandbeach Lake as a jumping-off point for some of the highest mountain summits in Rocky Mountain National Park.

DIRECTIONS: From the junction of US 36 and CO 7 in Estes Park, turn left on CO 7 and drive for 12.5 miles to Wild Basin Road, turn right and drive to the Rocky Mountain National Park Ranger Station. The Sandbeach Lake Trailhead is located immediately to the right of the kiosk. Go through the entrance and turn into the parking lot.

GPS Trailhead Coordinates   20 SANDBEACH LAKE TRAILHEAD: SANDBEACH LAKE

UTM zone (WGS84):   13T
Easting: 0454570
Northing: 4452070

SCENERY: ✿ ✿ ✿ ✿ ✿	DISTANCE: *9.8 miles out-and-back*
TRAIL CONDITION: ✿ ✿ ✿ ✿	HIKING TIME: *5 hours*
CHILDREN: ✿	OUTSTANDING FEATURES: *Waterfalls and*
DIFFICULTY: ✿ ✿ ✿ ✿	*water cascades: Copeland Falls, Calypso Cascades,*
SOLITUDE: ✿ ✿ ✿ ✿ ✿	*and Ouzel Falls; privacy, alpine lake*

The Ouzel Lake Campsite lies in a spruce–fir forest below the northeast slope of Copeland Mountain. You'd be hard pressed to find many people here or on the trail save for a few anglers above Calypso Cascades and a smattering of hikers. Constantly thundering waterfalls and cascades along the creeks, especially during spring runoff, are impressive sights and sounds you'll encounter along the entire route.

🏃 From the parking lot the trail immediately crosses a bridge over Hunters Creek. The trail is wide, fairly smooth, dirt, and level. Travel through lodgepole-pine trees and aspen trees. Less than a half mile from the trailhead is Copeland Falls, a sudden drop in North St. Vrain Creek. A social trail to the left of the main trail leads hikers to Copeland Falls. Take the detour to see both the upper and lower falls, and then rejoin the main trail.

After passing Copeland Falls, the trail narrows. Pass an intersection with a backcountry campsite trail and continue straight following the signs to Calypso Cascades and Ouzel Falls. Cross North St. Vrain Creek on a sturdy wood-and-stone bridge, complete with deafening falls in the springtime. Follow the trail uphill as it continues through the forest along Cony Creek to Calypso Cascades. This water feature is named for the namesake orchid that blooms here in July. Trails intersect at Calypso Cascades and hikers take a right turn, cross twin bridges, go around a bend, and cross a third bridge.

Remnants of damage from a well-known forest fire in 1978 can be seen from this point in the hike. Enough time has past since the Ouzel Fire that shrubs and flowers are plentiful in spot-burn areas.

For now, the water remains in the rearview mirror, making for a quieter ride. Climb a series of wide switchbacks and glimpse at the views of the surrounding mountain peaks. From right to left, the first peak is the south side of Mount Meeker with a good view of its knife-edge ridge along the top. Next to that is the south side of Longs Peak. A glance to the left and you will see a tremendous amount of downed timber and small landslides up on the hillside.

The distant sounds of the waterfalls are a constant reminder of the water in this area. Be patient since an uphill climb and more switchbacks are required before the next water views. Ouzel Falls is next, and it ranks as one of the most popular falls in Rocky Mountain National Park. Cross the trail's bridge spanning Ouzel Creek. Stop in the middle of the bridge to see the upper part of the falls which is a sheer drop. A great resting point will greet you a minute or two later with expansive views to the east. There is a really nice rock outcropping to sit on.

After crossing Ouzel Creek, the trail circles below the ridge where Ouzel Falls drops. Switchbacks wind downhill through boulders and under an overhanging cliff. At the next trail junction, take a left and continue to Ouzel Lake. This is Bluebird Lake Trail and it climbs to a crest, then becomes relatively straight and level; also, more narrow and rocky. This next section is extremely exposed, definitely not where you want to be during a storm. The views to the right are Tanima Peak and Mount Alice.

At the next trail intersection, take a left turn onto the spur to the Ouzel Lake Campsite. Wind downhill and rejoin Ouzel Creek. Travel along the creek until you see the outhouse for the Ouzel Lake Campsite. The campsite is just before Ouzel Lake, so if you've reached the lake, you've gone too far. Climb the stairs, pass the outhouse, proceed 150 feet, and you will be at the official tent site. A small trail continues west of the campsite, joins with the main trail, and leads to Ouzel Lake and a bear-proof container where campers can store their food for the night.

Ouzel Lake itself is dominated by Copeland Mountain. Ouzel and Manaha peaks are the other beauties visible from the lake. After a restful night, get up and go back the way that you came.

DIRECTIONS: From Estes Park and the junction of US 36 and CO 7, drive south on CO 7 via Marys Lake Road for 12.5 miles to the Wild Basin Road. Turn right and drive past the Wild Basin Inn and take the right-hand fork to the Entrance Station. Travel another 3 miles to the Ranger Station and Wild Basin Trailhead.

GPS Trailhead Coordinates	21 WILD BASIN TRAILHEAD: OUZEL LAKE CAMPSITE
UTM zone (WGS84):	13T
Easting:	0451970
Northing:	4450730

Northwest Side of Rocky Mountain National Park

Trail Ridge Road, Colorado River Headwaters Area, and Never Summer Range

Mo[...]
than 110
mountair[...]
peak[...]
towe[...]
ove[...]
the 415
squar[...]
miles o[...]
hiking
trails
picni[...]
spots
waterfalls
cold lakes
and
bountifu[...]
wildlife

22 Colorado River Trailhead:

Colorado River Trail to Lulu City

SCENERY: ✪ ✪ ✪ ✪	DISTANCE: *7.4 miles out-and-back*
TRAIL CONDITION: ✪ ✪ ✪ ✪	HIKING TIME: *3.5 hours*
CHILDREN: ✪ ✪ ✪	OUTSTANDING FEATURES: *Mining history,*
DIFFICULTY: ✪ ✪	*Colorado River, Never Summer Mountains, meadows*
SOLITUDE: ✪ ✪ ✪ ✪	

Lulu City is an old mining town that no longer exists, but the ghosts still linger. This trail maps the route to the town, passing old cabins and the mountain views the 200 or so residents would have seen in the late 1800s. The trail is level and follows the Colorado River with constant views of the mountain ridges of the Never Summers.

🚶 Leave the trailhead from the north side of the parking lot. The wide, dirt trail is shaded by large evergreen trees. Cross over a footbridge and officially enter Rocky Mountain National Park. Head up a set of deceiving switchbacks and get your blood moving. This little climb is deceiving because the majority of the trail is level or in a gradual ascent with only a total 200-foot elevation change to the turnaround point. There are man-made steps in the trail and just as quickly as you go up, you come down again.

To the left is the Colorado River. Cross two bridges, the first is a split log bridge and the second is a wider bridge. Reach the banks of the river, and the trail begins to travel along the river for a short time. There are many social trails that cut through to access the water.

The Colorado River conjures up visions of thundering rapids and towering canyons for most, but right here is the birthplace of the river. It's a great opportunity to see the waterway in a unique light, as a gurgling infant, calm and gentle, gathering up enough water to ebb and flow through the high country.

22 Colorado River Trailhead:
Colorado River Trail to Lulu City

N   0   1,500   3,000
feet

Lulu
City

Red Mtn. Trl.

Big Dutch Creek

Crater
Gulch

Shipler
Mtn.

SHIPLER
PARK
Cabins

Colorado River

ROCKY MTN.
NATIONAL PARK

Lost Creek

Squeak Creek

34

Opposition Creek

Phantom Creek

P

The landscape opens up for a short time along a small meadow. Reach a trail intersection at the edge of the meadow. Go straight here, continuing up the trail heading toward Shipler Cabins and Lulu City. At this point the trail begins a gradual ascent and narrows to a single-track, traversing above the river. The trail passes below an old rockslide; to the left are a meadow and new access to views of the surrounding peaks. Cross below another small rockslide; the trail is level here and easy to navigate as it proceeds north up the valley.

Pass a sign for Crater Creek, cross over it via a bridge, and continue. Shortly after Crater Creek, on the right, are the remains of the Shipler Cabins. These two tumbled log structures sit at the edge of Shipler Park—imagine the killer views they had, not to mention the killer winters! The trail continues to follow the stage road that ran through Lulu City and then northwest over mountain passes to Walden.

Cross a series of bridges and begin a gradual climb. The trail is again shaded by dense trees and views are lost, so is the access to the Colorado River. There are now roots sticking out of the dirt path, but it's still in great condition and easy to follow. As the trail ascends, a drop-off on the left side begins to develop, the forest gets very dense, and it becomes eerily quiet.

At the intersection with Little Yellowstone Canyon, Little Ditch, and La Poudre Pass, take a left on the trail headed downhill to Lulu City. Trail continues to descend with switchbacks, and a stream crossing, and then levels out again. A sign marks the Lulu City Site (1879–1884, population 200). Don't go looking for a ghost town, remarkable mining, or log cabin relics. The only memories here are written in the winds. From here, turn around and go back the way that you came.

DIRECTIONS: From the Grand Lake Entrance Station, take US 34 east for 9.6 miles. Turn left into the Colorado River Trailhead parking lot.

GPS Trailhead Coordinates	22 COLORADO RIVER TRAILHEAD: COLORADO RIVER TRAIL TO LULU CITY
UTM zone (WGS84):	13T
Easting:	0428040
Northing:	4479500

23 Corral Creek Trailhead:

Poudre River Trail to Cache Campsite

SCENERY: ✿ ✿ ✿ ✿ ✿	DISTANCE: *11.7 miles out–and–back*
TRAIL CONDITION: ✿	HIKING TIME: *6 hours*
CHILDREN: ✿ ✿	OUTSTANDING FEATURES: *Rivers, creeks,*
DIFFICULTY: ✿ ✿ ✿	*wildlife, high mountain peaks; unique access on*
SOLITUDE: ✿ ✿ ✿ ✿ ✿	*north side of Rocky Mountain National Park*

A better campsite couldn't be dreamed up. Cache Campsite is close to perfect. It is tucked into the trees at the edge of a mountain meadow in a high valley, surrounded by mountain peaks with a river running through it. This moderate 5.85-mile hike to Cache along the Cache la Poudre River is also a gem in its own right. There are open valleys and plentiful big game, especially deer and moose.

🚶 From the trailhead, proceed straight across the bridge. A sign indicates 1 mile to Rocky Mountain National Park boundary. The trail is an old double-track Jeep road in spots, single-track in others. Pass the boundary marker for Comanche Peak Wilderness. Head into a slight descent and follow the creek downstream. Pass wetlands, coniferous forests, and the intermittent views of the surrounding peaks. The trail is easy to follow.

Move quickly through the wetlands to avoid mosquitoes. Continue to follow La Poudre Pass Creek, which flows out of Long Draw Reservoir, downstream about a mile to its confluence with the Cache la Poudre River. The trail surface is soft dirt with occasional roots or rocks.

Bear right at the intersection with the Big South Trail. The Big South Trail heads north to CO 14 and has its own trailhead there.

Cross the bridge over the Cache la Poudre River, obviously bigger than La Poudre Pass Creek. At the time of the writing of this book, materials are on hand to build a large bridge here, including some big

23 Corral Creek Trailhead: **Poudre River Trail to Cache Campsite**

N

0   2,000   4,000
feet

COMANCHE PEAK WILDERNESS

Big South Trl.

Long Draw Rd.

To 14

La Poudre Pass Creek

Mummy Pass Trl.

Hague Creek

ROOSVEVELT NAT'L FOREST

Long Draw Reservoir

Cache la Poudre River

ROCKY MTN. NATIONAL PARK

Willow Creek

Chapin Creek Campsite

Cache Campsite

steel I beams, and we are not quite sure how they got here. Continue straight at the intersection with Mummy Pass Trail, following the signs to Chapin Creek. Immediately to the left is Hague Campsite, which I don't recommend since it's infested with mosquitoes.

This first half mile is extremely easy and follows the gentle grade of the river. Pay attention as the trail all but disappears in the wetland flats along the riverbank. Stay close to the river. When in doubt, remember that the trail eventually climbs up an embankment and away from the river. Hikers eventually come back near the river, looking down upon it as it cascades through a mini-gorge. Catch your breath and follow the trail uphill for a short steep ascent. Hike another mile and continue on trail as you emerge into a pristine valley. The trail is little worn through this valley, but easier to follow because the trees are not as dense. Pass any trail spurs or social trails and follow the trail up the valley. The trail climbs a small bluff, and the top is a great place to stop for views and a rest. Continue straight after descending from the little bluff.

The trail disappears but continues straight across the marshy area; continue to pay attention as the trail will veer right. Climb up into the woods, where carpetlike undergrowth covers the forest and your views are temporarily gone. The trail is very evident, so just follow it south. After a short descent, the trail is back down closer to river level. Travel a few hundred yards as the river bends off to the left and hikers continue straight, away from the river. Trail begins to ascend and becomes very obvious that you are on the right path. Exit the trees and enjoy the views of another large valley surrounded by mountain peaks.

Continue straight at an old sign indicating Chapin Creek Campsite to the left. Cache is straight ahead. The trail travels in and out of the trees, along the western edge of the meadow. The creek you can see now is Chapin Creek. As you walk along the edge of the valley, keep an eye out for the Cache Campground sign. It is easy to walk past. Signs indicate two separate tent sites. Both sit up in the trees. The campsite on the right is fairly spacious compared to most of the Rocky Mountain National Park backcountry sites. We camped here, and although it is in the trees, it is only 100 feet from the edge of the meadow. The campsite to the left is a little farther off the trail, not quite as large, but tucked better into the trees. Campers may wish to sit at the edge of the meadow as it gets dark and see who your neighbors are. When we camped, two moose came to call. Have fun camping and leave the way you came in the morning.

Take Note

ALTERNATE ACCESS

The Poudre Lake Trailhead, off Trail Ridge Road, is an alternate to the Poudre Canyon access. It gives hikers a 5.6-mile hike downhill to the Cache Campsite in Rocky Mountain National Park.

BACKCOUNTRY PERMIT

There is an information station, where you can get backcountry permits, at Corral Creek Trailhead; however, it isn't regularly staffed.

Hikers will need to plan ahead, pick up their backcountry permit in Rocky Mountain National Park at an earlier time and then head over to Poudre Canyon. (We did this and the Backcountry Office was very good about letting us pick up the backcountry permit on a separate trip to the park.)

TRAIL CONDITION

The first 1.5 miles of this trail are easy to follow. Then the trail travels through a series of open valleys and is not as easy to navigate. Some very wet areas and game trails will confuse you. The trail does go up and away from the river a few times but never for long. Just pay attention. When in doubt, keep traveling along the river and you will end up in the final and largest valley. That last section is where the hike skirts the trees, and you'll find Cache Campsite. You shouldn't get too lost here!

DIRECTIONS: From Fort Collins drive north on US 287 for 11 miles to CO 14. Turn left on CO 14 and follow it for 54 miles west to Long Draw Road. Turn left and travel 8.5 miles on Long Draw Road to the Corral Creek Trailhead on the left. On the other side of the road is an information cabin.

GPS Trailhead Coordinates	23 CORRAL CREEK TRAILHEAD: POUDRE RIVER TRAIL TO CACHE CAMPSITE
UTM zone (WGS84):	13T
Easting:	0434750
Northing:	4485330

SCENERY: ☆ ☆ ☆	DISTANCE: *1 mile out-and-back*
TRAIL CONDITION: ☆ ☆ ☆ ☆	HIKING TIME: *45 minutes*
CHILDREN: ☆ ☆ ☆ ☆ ☆	OUTSTANDING FEATURES: *Colorado River,*
DIFFICULTY: ☆	*Never Summer Mountains, wildlife, meadow*
SOLITUDE: ☆ ☆	

An easy trail that offers many rewards. Strollers and wheelchairs glide along without much effort through open meadow along the calm beginnings of the Colorado River. All hiking abilities can appreciate the views of the Never Summers, the informative signs, and promise of moose spotting. A great novice trail to get the youngsters interested in hiking. It's also a good one to keep the young-at-heart out on the trail.

🥾 Leave the parking area and travel to the trailhead kiosk. There are also restroom facilities here, adjacent to the parking area. The trail is packed dirt, mostly level, and is officially wheelchair accessible. Pass along a man-made fence and continue over a bridge that spans the Colorado River. The evergreen trees are dense and cooling at the trailhead, but once you cross the bridge the shade is left behind and replaced by meadowlands.

Take a right turn on the interpretive Coyote Valley Trail. To the left is a picnic area with a nicely spaced cluster of picnic tables in the trees. This area is for day use only, and there is no camping and no fires. Pass one of the many trail benches on the left. The trail continues to follow along the Colorado River. It's still completely level and flanked by thin stands of trees on the right. To the left are the meadows of the Kawuneeche Valley. When we hiked in the summer, the meadow was full of grass, browned by the sun, with patches of wildflowers peeking out.

The first interpretive sign hikers approach is of the riparian habitat. A colored line drawing shows representations of the water

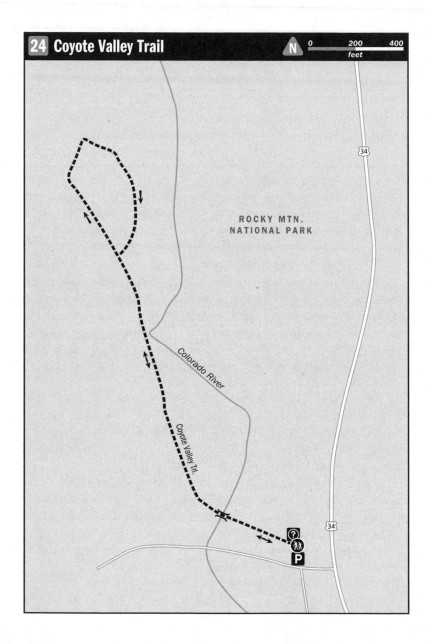

N

0   200   400
feet

34

ROCKY MTN.
NATIONAL PARK

Colorado River

Coyote Valley Trl.

34

shrew, the American dipper, and the chorus frog—all of whom are residents of this area.

Pass another man-made log bench and another and another and a small pond on the right. A number of benches line the route and offer a place to rest at almost any point in the trail. The trail begins to venture to cutbanks in the river. Social trails lead to the Colorado River shore. Pass three more interpretive signs: The Women of Life, The Visitors to the Kawuneeche, and The Mountain Meadows. Look straight ahead toward the mountains and spot the Grand Ditch. This large, roadlike cut in the mountainside is a horizontal line that traces early efforts to divert precious water from the Never Summers to other areas.

At the beginning of the balloon for the Coyote Valley Trail, go straight, traveling left along the west edge of the trail. This area offers a little more shade from the open meadow. The trail loops along and travels close to the river. It's easy to spot moose in this area because the marshy areas offer cool respites for the moose having their long, afternoon rests.

The Never Summers are in full view as the trail loops around. The larger peak is Baker Mountain, elevation 12,397 feet.

An interpretive sign speaks of a glacier valley that existed in this area. A sheet of ice, almost 20 miles long, once existed from the head of the Kawuneeche Valley, south to Shadow Mountain Lake. Only the highest peaks visible around rose 1,500 feet above the thick layer of ice as it carved this U-shaped valley. When the glacier receded, it left behind huge mounds of rock debris called moraines. Forests now grow in these ridges of rubble around the valley sides. Remnants of glacial ice still occupy the east-facing peaks high in the Never Summers to the left, or right, depending where you are in the loop.

The balloon is short and sweet, so get back on the trail and return by the same route. Stop at the picnic area on the way out, or skip rocks in the river.

DIRECTIONS: From the Grand Lake Entrance Station, take US 34 east 5.6 miles to the Coyote Valley Trailhead. Turn left onto the access road and dead end at the parking lot.

GPS Trailhead Coordinates	24 COYOTE VALLEY TRAIL
UTM zone (WGS84):	13T
Easting:	0427128
Northing:	4466139

25 Holzwarth Historic Site:

Never Summer Ranch

SCENERY: ☆ ☆ ☆
TRAIL CONDITION: ☆ ☆ ☆ ☆
CHILDREN: ☆ ☆ ☆ ☆ ☆
DIFFICULTY: ☆
SOLITUDE: ☆ ☆

DISTANCE: *1.14 miles out–and–back*
HIKING TIME: *45 minutes*
OUTSTANDING FEATURES: *Colorado River, Never Summer Mountains, meadow, historic buildings, nature walk*

The colorful history of this amazing little ranch is enough for any hiker to long for the old days. Whether it's the rustic tourist complex created in 1920 (Holzwarth Trout Lodge) or the guest and dude ranch that operated into the 1970s (Never Summer Ranch), you'll wish you would have stayed here. The trail is level and mostly accessible by strollers or wheelchairs. The buildings, however, are not handicap accessible.

🏃🏃 Begin from the parking area which accesses the flat, glacially carved Kawuneeche Valley at the foot of the Never Summer Mountains. The rustic buildings that still exist are the final destination on this hike and offer a glimpse into the history of the pioneers at the turn of the 20th century. One of the cabins is located right at the trailhead and was built by a neighboring homesteader and miner. The cabin is equipped on most summer weekend days with a knowledgeable volunteer. All buildings on this hike are open daily from 10 a.m. to 4 p.m., and there are restrooms at the trailhead.

Leave the trailhead cabin and follow the dirt road toward the river and the trees. The trail is a level dirt road. Continue across the valley, looking left down the Kawuneeche Valley. Interpretive signs throughout the path tell hikers of the Never Summer Ranch.

One of the Kawuneeche Valley's first dude ranches once thrived here. In 1917 German immigrants Sophia and John Holzwarth built their homestead here after wartime prohibition closed their saloon

25 Holzwarth Historic Site:
Never Summer Ranch

N

0   208   416
feet

34

Cabin

Ditch Rd.

Colorado River

ROCKY MTN.
NATIONAL PARK

Holzwarth
Cabins

in Denver. Originally, ranchers began hosting friends from the city at the Holzwarth Trout Lodge. More visitors followed. The Never Summer Ranch, as it was later known, offered fishing, hunting, and horseback rides. Guests stayed in rustic cabins or a lodge that once stood in the meadow before us.

In 1975, Never Summer Ranch and Holzwarth Homestead became part of Rocky Mountain National Park. Although the newer buildings were removed to restore the meadow, this dirt road leads to the Holzwarth original homestead buildings. In its historic heyday, the Never Summer Ranch offered horseback riding, hunting, and all the trout you could catch for $2 a day or $11 a week.

The infantile Colorado River flows to the right, where at a mere 10 miles upstream it begins, in a trickle to the Pacific watershed. Pass interpretive signs about moose, which are plentiful in this area. Cross the Colorado River via a bridge. Pass old farm equipment and fence posts, which look like the outline of an old corral. Continue on the road and head into an area that is a little more shaded thanks to the evergreen trees that mark the beginning of the ranch.

The first signs appear: HOLZWARTH TROUT LODGE, 1920–29, and before you know it, you've made it to the destination. Take time to circle around and tour the buildings. Included are a taxidermy shop, kitchens, bunk house, ice house, wood shed, old sleds, wagons, and more. If you try really hard, you may even be able to smell the bacon that Sophia may have been frying up on a cool summer morning. Then close your eyes and dream of the rugged simplicity that characterized the West when it was young. After a look at the historic site, turn around and head back the way you came.

DIRECTIONS: From the Grand Lake Entrance Station, take US 34 east 7.2 miles to the sign for Holzwarth Historic Site. Turn left into the parking lot.

GPS Trailhead Coordinates	25 HOLZWARTH HISTORIC SITE: NEVER SUMMER RANCH
UTM zone (WGS84):	13T
Easting:	0427479
Northing:	4469263

26 Milner Pass Trailhead: *Continental Divide Trail to Mount Ida*

SCENERY: ☆ ☆ ☆ ☆	DISTANCE: *10 miles out-and-back*
TRAIL CONDITION: ☆ ☆ ☆	HIKING TIME: *6 hours*
CHILDREN: ☆ ☆	OUTSTANDING FEATURES: *Alpine tundra,*
DIFFICULTY: ☆ ☆ ☆ ☆	*bighorn sheep, elk, summer tundra wildflowers,*
SOLITUDE: ☆ ☆ ☆ ☆	*expansive views, Continental Divide*

The summit of Mount Ida is accessed via a tundra trek that travels along the crest of the Continental Divide. Solitude is a guarantee here as are the promises of incredible scenery and the chance to see plenty of wildlife. Once at the summit, there is an equal reward waiting with views of the alpine basin of the Gorge Lakes. Most of the hike is above tree line in open tundra. This is cause for advance planning; leave early and be willing to turn back if you spot developing storms.

Milner Pass Trailhead is a busy place, so exit quickly and head toward Poudre Lake, a small beaver pond to the left of the parking area. Travel along the Old Fall River Road and the Ute Trail, also an official Continental Divide Landmark. Begin to ascend, switchback, and travel up the stairs. Pass rock spires along the left as the trail continues to switchback and travel along a ridge. There is still traffic noise from Trail Ridge Road, but due to the quick ascent of the trail, you travel away from the crowds very quickly.

The trail levels out for a little bit, but makes sure that you still do sufficient huffing and puffing. Cross a split-log bridge over a dry gully and then continue onward and upward. At the trail junction, approximately a mile from the trailhead, continue straight following the sign that says MOUNT IDA. The large switchback, which goes up the left, takes other hikers toward the Alpine Visitor Center and the Old Fall River Road.

Milner Pass
Trailhead

*Poudre
Lake*

34

P

**Sheep
Rock**

**ROCKY MTN.
NATIONAL PARK**

Continental Divide Nat'l Scenic Trl.

**Jacksaw
Mtn.**

*Larimer County
Grand County*

*Timber
Lake*

**Mt.
Ida**

*Inkwell
Lake*

*Azure
Lake*

Look to your right in the southwest direction for views of the
Never Summer Mountains. The trail begins a descent, making this
section of trail much easier. It continues to stay easy as the trail
follows a level path through a marshy area and then crosses a split-log
bridge.

With the marshy conditions there may be spots of mud. When we
hiked in midsummer, we spotted a lot of animal tracks crisscrossing
the muddy sections. Rock steps signal the start of your next climbing
segment—so much for restful hiking on easy terrain. The trees become
dense as this trail continues a milder grade uphill. It is here that we
spotted a giant elk with a 12-point antler rack.

Traverse around the hill and begin to walk right through the
tundra and you crest at 11,379 feet. After we had traversed along the
western ridge on our hike, we came upon a group of bighorn sheep—
four lambs and eight adults. This also looks like a spot where the
sheep bed down, since the tundra grass appears to be matted down.

Now begins the long, hard trek above timberline, complete with
large traverses, switchbacks, and a lot of false summits. You think
you've reached Mount Ida, then you look across and there it is again.

Continue on, and if the trail becomes faint, follow the cairns, always heading uphill, in a southern trajectory. You'll be required in spots to scramble over easy boulder fields in the midst of the tundra to reach the summit of Mount Ida at 12,880 feet. From here you see views of Chief Cheley Peak, Cracktop, Mount Julian, and Terra Tomah Mountain. The shimmering waters below form the Gorge Lakes drainage. From here, at a 2,000-foot elevation gain from 10,745 feet, turn around and head back the way that you came.

DIRECTIONS: From the Grand Lake Entrance Station, take US 34 east 16 miles to the Milner Pass Trailhead. Turn right into the parking lot.

GPS Trailhead Coordinates	26 MILNER PASS TRAILHEAD: CONTINENTAL DIVIDE TRAIL TO MOUNT IDA
UTM zone (WGS84):	13T
Easting:	0431210
Northing:	4474520

5

Southwest Side of Rocky Mountain National Park

Tonahutu Area,
East Inlet Area and
North Inlet Area

More
than 110
mountain
peaks
tower
over
the 415
square
miles of
hiking
trails
picnic
spots
waterfalls
cold lakes
and
bountiful
wildlife

SCENERY: ☆ ☆ ☆ ☆ ☆	DISTANCE: *13.8 miles out-and-back*
TRAIL CONDITION: ☆ ☆ ☆	HIKING TIME: *8 hours*
CHILDREN: ☆	OUTSTANDING FEATURES: *Creeks, lakes,*
DIFFICULTY: ☆ ☆ ☆ ☆	*waterfalls, optimum chance of seeing moose; views of*
SOLITUDE: ☆ ☆ ☆ ☆ ☆	*numerous mountain peaks including Mt. Alice and*
	Mt. Craig

After the first few easy miles, all with a high probability of seeing moose, the trail becomes steep and takes hikers to a wonderful wooded campsite on a spectacular subalpine lake: Lake Verna. This overnight destination is unique because it's ringed by high alpine peaks, and the campsite itself is the highest elevation of all the campsites on this trial. Lake Verna also signifies the end of the maintained trail; the trail does continue, but it's not maintained by Rocky Mountain National Park.

🚶 The East Portal Trailhead shares a parking lot with the public boat launch. Don't be confused. Instead, leave the trailhead and get on the trail by crossing through a small sagebrush meadow. Cross over a bridge that protects hikers from a low, marshy area and enter into a lodgepole-pine forest. Many of the trees here are brownish red because they have been killed by pine beetles.

Pass the spur trail to Adams Falls. Proceed up the rock stairs, which are half naturally placed and half man-laid. The trail is single-track and hard-packed dirt. A minute or two after you pass another entrance to Adams Falls and the Adams Falls Loop, hikers begin to travel along a small creek.

Don't be discouraged by the damage to the lodgepole pines. On this particular trail, nature has begun to take its restorative course and aspen trees are already filling in the areas vacated by the lodgepole pine.

Andrews
Peak

Lake Verna
Campsite

Lake Verna

East Inlet Creek

Lone
Pine
Lake

Mt.
Craig

TEN LAKE
PARK

Lower East Inlet
Campground

Mt.
Cairns

Mt.
Wescott

ROCKY MTN.
NATIONAL PARK

East
Meadow
Campsite

Portal Rd.

To 34

Adams
Falls

Mt.
Bryant

There are always many day hikers on the first few miles of this trail, and it isn't rare to pass groups with no daypacks or even water supplies. If these hikers ask how far it is to Lake Verna, be sure to tell them that it's almost seven miles. That way, they won't be disillusioned by the ease of the first part of the trail. When we hiked, we passed a hiker with a walker. When we returned the next day, the walker had been abandoned a few miles from the trailhead. Peculiar.

Pass alongside wetlands, an open meadow full of grasses, and views of the mountain peaks ahead. Continue to follow the trail along the north side of this meadow. The trail will pass through the wetlands for sometime. This gives hikers ample opportunity to see moose since they frequent this area.

The trail beings to climb slowly above those meadows, so there are plenty of opportunities for different vantage points and moose viewing. Pass the turnoffs for the East Meadow campsites. A sign here encourages hikers to stay on the main trail and go 100 yards beyond the turnoff for what the park service calls a "prime moose-viewing overlook with wetlands, meadow views, and everything right in front of you." As predicted, when we hiked, there was a moose walking on the far end of the meadow. They are easily recognized because they are dark brown, the size of a large horse, with long legs and a unique walk. There is also no mistaking the moose that have the trademark plate antlers.

Follow the trail as it climbs into the woods across a tiny, rustic, split-log bridge. This portion of the trail seems to come alive because of the diversity of the trees—spruce, fir, and pine—that reach toward the sky.

One hundred yards later is a longer split-log bridge. When crossing, look for a small waterfall coming off the rocks to the left. A few minutes of climbing will bring you to your next bridge, a little more formal and constructed in style. Also, there is a great view of the rock formations above.

From this point forward, the wildlife viewing and easy hiking are over. As the trail gets steeper past the Lower East Inlet campsite, look for a nice rock on your right to rest. After that rock is a very rocky, steep section with a large rock on your left and a drop-off on your right. This is an unforgiving point on the path, and it will not let you forget that you have a pack on.

Follow the steep and narrow single-track trail as it continues up along the left-hand wall of this valley.

The valley has slowly narrowed into a gorge. The trail begins to switchback, traveling to the north and then northwest. Wind through the boulders and up the steep man-made rock stairs. A set of down-hill stairs follows, as hikers head back toward the creek. Take in the view and the falls and then, just past the falls is a great place to take off your boots and cool your feet in the creek.

The next mile is uneventful. Then hikers come to an area where part of the bark has been removed from some trees near the ground. As I watch, a squirrel is completely debarking a tree up at the top, and it's raining bark on me.

Cross another split-log bridge and look to the left where another beautiful waterfall is coming down the face of a rock. Continue on, and eventually views of higher peaks come into frame. Cross a wood-and-stone bridge over East Inlet Creek. We are 9,500 feet above sea level here. There are 780 feet and approximately 2 miles left to hike. The next destination is Lone Pine Lake. Hike along the south side of the lake, then cross a nice series of bridges. The first two have waterfalls. The trail continues to climb, and the surface is well maintained though very rocky. The last mile in the approach to the campsite is surprisingly easy. It travels along the creek and then eventually passes a hitching rail. Take a left onto the small trail that leads uphill to the Lake Verna campsite. So, now you are at your stop for the night and at Lake Verna. The campsite itself is only a small clearing in the forest with space for your tent and a separate cooking area. You may want to spend your time at the beautiful area below your campsite on the shore of Lake Verna. Have a good rest, and in the morning head back the way you came.

DIRECTIONS: From the Grand Lake Entrance Station, take US 34 west 1.6 miles and turn left into Grand Lake Village; stay on the left fork, West Portal Road, and travel 2.4 miles to the East Inlet Trailhead.

GPS Trailhead Coordinates	27 EAST INLET TRAILHEAD: LAKE VERNA CAMPSITE
UTM zone (WGS84):	13T
Easting:	0431920
Northing:	4454420

Mountain Lake and Ranger Meadows Balloon

SCENERY: ☆ ☆ ☆ ☆	DISTANCE: *6 miles, balloon*
TRAIL CONDITION: ☆ ☆ ☆ ☆	HIKING TIME: *2.5 hours*
CHILDREN: ☆ ☆ ☆ ☆	OUTSTANDING FEATURES: *Shadow*
DIFFICULTY: ☆ ☆	*Mountain Lake, Colorado River, creeks, meadows,*
SOLITUDE: ☆ ☆ ☆ ☆	*lake scenery*

This will be a favorite trail. If not for the beauty of the forested landscape along the lake or the tall grasses and wildflowers of Ranger Meadows, you will be most impressed by the lack of other hikers and the pristine paths. The trail crosses the boundary between Rocky Mountain National Park and the National Forest Service; a difference between the two is not significant.

🏃 Leave the parking lot and walk across the spillway of Shadow Mountain Dam. To the left is Shadow Mountain Lake, and to the right is the water being let loose from the lake into the Colorado River, which then flows into Columbine Bay.

Reach the East Shore Trailhead and take a left onto the trail that enters Rocky Mountain National Park in 0.6 miles. The trail travels along a ridge on the east side of Shadow Mountain Lake. This section of the trail provides wonderful, scenic views out over the water. The trail surface is level, mostly packed dirt, and continues to follow the shore until it turns away from the lake at a gentle ascent and then continues into the forest.

The trail travels back around toward the lake. It's lush in spots, marshy and muddy in others. Continue straight past the first intersection, 2 miles from the East Shore Trailhead. The trail rises up above the lake. Pass a sign that says ENTERING ROCKY MOUNTAIN NATIONAL PARK, SHADOW MOUNTAIN LOOKOUT 4.8 MILES AND SHADOW

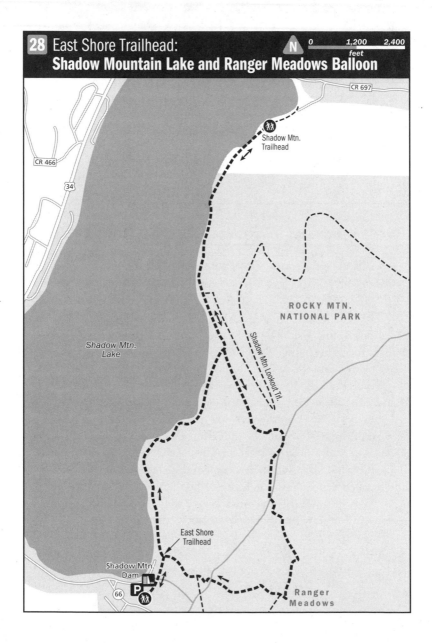

28 East Shore Trailhead:
Shadow Mountain Lake and Ranger Meadows Balloon

N

0   1,200   2,400
feet

CR 697

CR 466

34

Shadow Mtn.
Trailhead

ROCKY MTN.
NATIONAL PARK

Shadow Mtn.
Lake

Shadow Mtn Lookout Trl.

East Shore
Trailhead

Shadow Mtn.
Dam

66

Ranger
Meadows

MOUNTAIN DAM 2.8 MILES. The Shadow Mountain Lookout Trail is a strenuous trek to a unique, historic fire lookout. Continue to the Shadow Mountain Trailhead on the north side of the hike and turn around. Trace back the trail that you have already traveled.

Pass the Shadow Mountain Lookout sign again and head back to the next intersection where hikers turn left onto Outlet Trail and head to Ranger Meadows. Cross over Ranger Creek where the trail is overgrown with meadow grasses. Continue through the meadow, keeping an eye out for moose. The meadow and the trail skirt in and out of the edge of the forest.

At the next trail intersection, turn right up the hill following the directions to East Shore Trail and Shadow Mountain Dam. Cross over a marshy bog that is covered by long, split-log double bridges and then comes back out on the trail. The last intersection is back to the East Shore Trailhead, traveling along the Colorado River, climbing up the right side of the dam. Head left, back across the dam, and back to the parking lot.

DIRECTIONS: From the Grand Lake Entrance Station, take US 34 west past the Grand Lake Village for 2.8 miles to a left turn into Green Ridge Complex (CO 66). Travel 1 mile, and make a left turn into the campground. Drive up toward the lake and turn right into the next campground and park at the Shadow Mountain Dam. Pay the U.S. Forest Service fee at Shadow Mountain Dam.

GPS Trailhead Coordinates	28 EAST SHORE TRAILHEAD: SHADOW MOUNTAIN LAKE AND RANGER MEADOWS BALLOON
UTM zone (WGS84):	13T
Easting:	0428440
Northing:	4450700

Creek Trail to Renegade Campsite to Flattop Mountain

SCENERY: ✿ ✿ ✿ ✿ ✿	DISTANCE: *23.2 miles out-and-back to Flattop*
TRAIL CONDITION: ✿ ✿ ✿	*Mountain (14.6 miles out-and-back to Renegade*
CHILDREN: ✿	*Campsite) 16 miles thru-hike (Green Mountain*
DIFFICULTY: ✿ ✿ ✿ ✿	*Trailhead to Bear Lake Trailhead)*
SOLITUDE: ✿ ✿ ✿ ✿	HIKING TIME: *13 hours out-and-back to*
	Flattop Mountain (8 hours out-and-back to
	Renegade Campsite) 9 hours for thru-hike (Green
	Mountain Trailhead to Bear Lake Trailhead)
	OUTSTANDING FEATURES: *Meadows, forest,*
	timberline, tundra, waterfall, creek

This is a rare hike that traverses the Continental Divide and takes hikers from the west side of Rocky Mountain National Park to the east side. Renegade is a good stopping point and an even better campsite. There are plenty of options in this hike; the first is a start at Green Mountain Trailhead, camp at Renegade, hike to Flattop Mountain, and then turn around. If you want to hike to Renegade, camp, and then turn around, that's great, too. A final option is to hike from Green Mountain Trailhead to Bear Lake Trailhead. This requires arranging a shuttle ride from either trailhead.

    🚶🚶 From the parking lot, leave the trailhead and start on the 1.8-mile uphill trek to Big Meadow. The first part of the trail is wide, packed dirt, and very easy to navigate albeit quite steep. The trail then moderates for the remaining mile to Big Meadow. Cross a number of large wooden bridges and pass several meadows through the trees on the right. Each meadow is progressively bigger than the one before it. A short downhill brings hikers to the largest meadow, living up to its name: Big Meadow.

    At the intersection of Green Mountain Trail and Tonahutu Creek Trail, take a left turn. Follow the trail along the north side of

29 Green Mtn. Trailhead: **Tonahutu Creek**
Trail to Renegade Campsite to Flattop Mtn.

N

| 0 | 0.85 | 1.7 |

miles

Marguerite
Falls

Bear
Lake

Hallett
Peak

Notchtop
Mtn.

Little
Matterhorn

Flattop
Mtn.

Knobtop
Mtn.

Bighorn
Flats

Stones
Peak

Sprague
Mtn.

Sprague
Glacier

Continental Divide National Scenic Trl.

Snowdrift
Peak

Larimer County

Grand County

Renegade
Campsite

Granite
Falls

Nakai
Peak

ROCKY MTN.
NATIONAL PARK

Onahu Creek

Green
Mtn.

P

34

Big Meadow. There are remnants of an old cabin to the left and more cabin remnants farther along the trail to the right. Your destination, Flattop Mountain, is not visible at this point, although other high peaks have come into view.

Take the trail north and then curve east along the far end of Big Meadow. Big Meadow is about a mile long. At the intersection of Tonahutu Creek Trail and Onahu Creek Trail, bear right, staying on Tonahutu Creek Trail. Then head back into the trees, heading in an easterly direction all the way to the campsite.

After a quarter mile hiking into the trees, hikers come to Tonahutu Creek, which flows along the trail for a while. Pass Sunset and Sunrise campsites on the left. There is a slight grade in the trail and then it levels off. This is a pleasant walk in the woods with nothing of great note, and then the trail is abruptly interrupted by a steep rock section and very steep stairs above them. At the top of that short section, Lower Granite Falls Campsite is to the right. A few minutes later, another steep section marks a change in this hike, a change that makes this hike more difficult.

After the steep, rocky section, the trail comes to Granite Falls, a two-tiered water cascade over the rocks. Take a break near the rocks at the base of the falls. Another extremely steep section brings hikers to Granite Falls Campsite on the left. Cross over the bridge and cross a large meadow that offers new views of the surrounding mountain peaks.

Tonahutu Creek's water thunders along the trail through here. Keep hiking through the trees on the rocky trail. Arrive at Tonahutu Meadows and Tonahutu Meadows Campsites on the east end of the meadow. Pass the intersection to the trail that goes downhill to the Tonahutu Stock Campsite. Be sure to go uphill to the left of this intersection.

It's pretty obvious that these campsites are responsible for a lot of the use of the trail up to this point. The trail we are on is much smaller and lesser traveled now. It is still steep, the creek tumbling along down the side of us. Cross the creek and pass the Haynach Campsite.

Some of these trees are quite large for being right below timberline. There is a sharp left in the trail and in 100 feet, hikers will see the sign for Renegade Campsite on the left. A few hundred feet up the trail is the silver arrow marking the campsite and the designation where campers are supposed to camp within 15 feet of this silver arrow. Although a little slanted, this site is a little bit bigger and more open than the usual area for your tent at a backcountry site. The trees are large but well spaced. There are views of the surrounding peaks, through the trees. This will be our stop for the night. Paths lead off to the left to another possible campsite, although not within the 15 feet of the silver arrow. There are rocks and stumps around for sitting and setting up camp.

In the morning, go back down to the main trail and take a left turn. Continue up the hill. In a few minutes, you will be in the shadow of Sprague Mountain, hiking toward an old rockslide. As we get in front of the rockslide, the trail makes an abrupt curve to the right.

Pass the turnoff to Timberline Campsite, a group site, to the left. Cross a split-log bridge and come to a warning sign. This is a posting of a 3-D map of what is to come in the trail—basically a warning that this trail goes through Bighorn Flats for several miles above tree line. There is severe weather with snow whiteouts, even in summer. Hikers can easily loose their way in the snow or the fog.

The trail takes a right and crosses debris at the base of the rockslide. Continue up; views from this point are tremendous with snow-covered peaks across the valley to the right. The trail is extremely rough and rocky; continue to follow it through the car-sized boulders and back into the tress. Even in late summer, water will be flowing down the trail during this section. Over your right shoulder is Nakai Peak, which is also visible from the other direction down in Big Meadow. The traverse you are starting lasts about three-quarters of a mile. You'll cross numerous little creeks and streams. After a quarter mile you will come out of the forest proper. There are still some stands of trees ahead but nothing much, and the trail goes up over the top of the ridge.

You will begin to see rock cairns at this point. You may notice a few points above you on the traverse where there are some little used switchbacks that are extremely steep and hard to follow. This is not the trail and not where we want to go. After a stand of trees, the trail climbs a little bit and continues across the tundra. Snow off to the right commands much of the view. A raised level mountain that you that see in front of us is not Flattop Mountain, just a false summit.

We continue to cross Bighorn Flats through open tundra for quite a while (about 2 miles). Frequent cairns, often only 100 yards apart, guide hikers as we head to the northern shoulder of Bighorn Flats. Storm Peak comes into view over your left shoulder and Knobtop Mountain is the next landmark in front of us. The trail veers to the south for a half mile and back east toward Ptarmigan Point, the knobby protrusion in front of you.

From the trail you can see the Grand Valley. The grade here is extremely mild, and walking is very easy, even though we've been

DAY & OVERNIGHT HIKES

WEST SIDE OF RMNP

part five

SOUTHWEST SIDE OF RMNP

traveling above 12,000 feet for quite a while now. Keep heading straight up the top of Bighorn Flats. There are very few turns here but enough marmots to keep you occupied.

As you get below the rocky crag in front of us, trail veers southwest, going a little bit to the right. Hikers can see Grand Lake and Shadow Mountain Lake clearly all of a sudden, way, way down the mountain. Trail veers on the right side of Ptarmigan Point and goes back east again for half a mile to Flattop Mountain. From this side, Flattop Mountain is a terminus of Bighorn Flats; it's more rugged on the other side. Hallett Peak is directly in front of you and stands at 12,713 feet, making it now the nearest and most prominent landmark. We now head toward it.

You can see the trail straight ahead and visibility is good for a long time. There is a very rugged view beyond that and rugged drop-offs coming into view to the left. Go around Ptarmigan Point, and the trail actually goes downhill before going back up to the top of Flattop Mountain. If the weather is good, go over to the viewpoint on the left just before Flattop Mountain. There are tremendous views looking down to three lakes that lie below.

This is not a good place to wander off the trail if visibility is bad. In Bighorn Flats it was fairly safe, but from here on, there are some tremendous drop-offs to the left. From the overlook it's back uphill at a mild grade. Pass the intersection with North Inlet Trail and continue straight up the hill. Next stop is the top of Flattop Mountain.

From here you can turn around and go back to Renegade Campsite for the night and then back to the Green Mountain Trailhead. Or you can head east down to the Bear Lake Trailhead.

DIRECTIONS: From the Grand Lake Entrance Station, take US 34 east 2.8 miles to the Green Mountain Trailhead. Turn right into the parking lot.

GPS Trailhead Coordinates	29 GREEN MOUNTAIN TRAILHEAD: TONAHUTU CREEK TRAIL TO RENEGADE CAMPSITE TO FLATTOP MOUNTAIN
UTM zone (WGS84):	13T
Easting:	0428560
Northing:	4461960

Creek Trail and Green Mountain Trail Loop

SCENERY: ✫ ✫ ✫ ✫	DISTANCE: *7.6 miles, loop*
TRAIL CONDITION: ✫ ✫ ✫ ✫	HIKING TIME: *4 hours*
CHILDREN: ✫ ✫ ✫	OUTSTANDING FEATURES: *Loop hike, Big*
DIFFICULTY: ✫ ✫ ✫	*Meadow, Onahu Creek, homesteader remnants,*
SOLITUDE: ✫ ✫ ✫ ✫	*lodgepole-pine forest, aspen trees, a lot of shade*

Alas, a long loop hike in Rocky Mountain National Park. Believe me, loop day hikes are hard to come by in the park. This hike is a quiet walk in the woods, with only the "creaking" of fallen lodgepole pines to break your concentration and give you a little spook. By combining Onahu Creek, Tonahutu and Green Mountain trails, you form a circle through some amazing scenery. This is a long, uncrowded walk with a variety of creeks, streams, cascades, aspen trees, and more. Be sure to bring along a buddy and plenty of supplies.

🚶🚶 Leave the Onahu Creek Trailhead, taking a left turn onto the trail. It's a 6.9-mile trek to the Green Mountain Trailhead and then another 0.7 miles to make it back to this trailhead.

The first destination to set your sights on is the Onahu Bridge, which is 3 miles from the trailhead.

The trail travels along the edge of Trail Ridge Road at first; it's level, dirt, single-tracked, and, in the summer, lined with grasses and wildflowers. The trail begins to turn away from the road and travels at a slight ascent through meadow and forest mix.

As you travel deeper into the forest, the trees become dense and ferns cover the moist ground. There are many fallen trees here, and they begin to give off their customary creaking sound as any sort of breeze settles in. It's almost reminiscent of an old door being opened

N

0   1,350   2,700
feet

Onahu Creek

ROCKY MTN.
NATIONAL PARK

Tonahutu
Creek Trl.

Onahu Creek
Trailhead

P

34

Green Mtn.
Trailhead

in a haunted house. You'll find yourself looking over your shoulder more than once.

Pass through a few gentle switchbacks and continue through a small aspen grove. The trail then makes a moderate descent as it passes through aspens that have been scratched and scarred by animals.

Continue to meander up and down in roller-coaster fashion. So far, the trail has been quite mossy, and when we hiked in midsummer, there were a lot of bugs, mosquitoes primarily, and trees full of mossy lichen.

Begin another small descent, while approaching a small stream. Cross the water on a split-log bridge and then travel up again to where the trail levels out and follows a hillside in a long, deep switchback. The trail levels out again and enters the dense forest. Begin another climb along a hillside, where to your left you will hear and then see a cascading waterfall.

The next waypoint is Onahu Creek, which we've been traveling along for a while now. Cross over it on a stout bridge and begin to travel upward again. Come back around toward the creek and cross another bridge, spanning a stream that feeds into Onahu Creek.

The trail continues to travel uphill with the sound of Onahu Creek on the right. It then levels out and travels along a flat forested area. There are many rocks and trees in the path. Pass the signs that direct backpackers to backcountry campsites: Onahu Creek, Upper Onahu, and Onahu Bridge. On the right through the tress a large meadow opens up. The trail is still level and has gotten softer and sandier. The trail starts to go uphill again and continues alongside Onahu Creek on the right. Stay on task and take the Onahu Bridge to cross over Onahu Creek. Continue past the next sign toward the Tonahutu Creek Trail, 1.5 miles. The climb resumes, continuing uphill and passing through a rockslide of large boulders.

The trail travels up a steep ledge and to the right is a big drop-off. The trail levels out for a short while. The trail is fairly level and then begins a gradual descent. The trail is narrower now, and if you look to the left you can see a tree-covered mountain ridge come into view. Pass the trail intersection with Flattop Mountain and Bear Lake. Onahu Creek Trailhead is 4.5 miles behind you. Continue straight. After passing that intersection, you will come upon Big Meadow on the left. A few minutes walk along the meadow and you will pass an old homestead and cabin remnants. It's a testament to Sam Stone's taste for views. He was the original homesteader on this property in the early 1900s.

At the end of Big Meadow, pass a hitch rack; you will also pass Big Meadow Campsite on your left. We will take the main trail uphill to Green Mountain trailhead, 1.8 miles. The uphill is short and you have a long pleasant downhill. The path is wide, fairly smooth, and gently graded down to Green Mountain Trailhead. Pass several small meadows on your left through the trees. Cross a series of bridges over small creeks and then arrive at the Green Mountain Trailhead. From here, cross through the parking lot to the trail that will take you back to the Onahu Creek Trailhead. The short walk back to the original trailhead is through a small forest that travels alongside Trail Ridge Road.

DIRECTIONS: From the Grand Lake Entrance Station, take
US 34 east 3.3 miles to the Onahu Creek Trailhead. Turn right
into the parking lot.

GPS Trailhead Coordinates	30 ONAHU CREEK TRAILHEAD: ONAHU CREEK TRAIL AND GREEN MOUNTAIN TRAIL LOOP
UTM zone (WGS84):	13T
Easting:	0428670
Northing:	4462020

Appendix A: Camping-equipment Checklist

Summer Backpacking-gear Checklist

Backpack
Tent and rain fly
Sleeping bag and sleeping pad or mattress
Water filter or purification tablets
Water bottles
Flashlight—fresh and extra batteries
Candle lantern (optional)
Trowel or small shovel for digging "cat holes"
Pocketknife
Bear canister
50 feet of rope and nylon cord
Topographical map and GPS unit
Toilet paper and plastic bags for packing it out
Biodegradable hand soap
Toothbrush and toothpaste
Small towel
Bandannas
Whistle
Stuff sacks
Sewing kit
Food—including extra for emergencies
Cooking pots/pans—nesting
Eating utensils—cup, bowl, plate, knife, fork, spoon
Cleaning supplies—biodegradable detergent and container,

sponge, scouring pad
Waterproof matches in waterproof container
Stove and fuel
Collapsible bucket or water bag
Hat
Poncho or rain gear
Boots
Boot socks
Sock liners
Long pants
Shorts
Light shirt or T-shirt
Warm shirt
Jacket or outerwear (layer clothing)
Other clothing depending on conditions and altitude
Appropriate undergarments

First-aid Kit

Pain reliever
Band-Aids
First-aid cream
Gauze pads
Insect repellent
Moleskin
UV sunblock, lip balm
Personal medications
Adhesive tape

Appendix B: RMNP Backcountry Camping Guide

How to Get Your Permit

You must have a permit to camp overnight in RMNP's backcountry. You can pick one up at the Headquarters Backcountry Office or at the Kawuneeche Visitor Center.

To minimize impacts on the park's resources, the number of permits issued is limited. You may obtain day-of-trip permits in person year-round. You may make reservations by mail or in person anytime after March 1 for a permit for that calendar year. You may make reservations by phone from March 1 to May 15 and anytime after October 1 for a permit for that calendar year.

CONTACT INFORMATION:
Backcountry Permits
Rocky Mountain National Park
Estes Park, CO 80517
(970) 586-1242
TDD (for those who are hearing-impaired):
(970) 586-1319

FOR ALL RESERVATIONS:

1. Include your name, address, zip code, and telephone number.

2. List an itinerary with dates corresponding to campsites where you plan to stay.

3. Specify the number of people that will be in your party. (Limit of seven per party for individual campsites. Limit of 12 per party for group campsites.)

4. There is a $20 administrative fee for permits during peak season periods (nonrefundable). Fees are not to be sent when requesting reservations, but are payable (by cash or check only) when the permit is issued.

To assist you, a Backcountry Trip Planning Worksheet is available. Please mail it in or have it with you when making in-person or phone reservations.

During the winter and early spring when the backcountry is not as frequently used, you may self-register at the Wild Basin Winter Trailhead, Sandbeach Lake Trailhead, Longs Peak Ranger Station, Dunraven Trailhead, and Fall River and Beaver Meadows entrance stations.

During the busy summer months, if you have a permit reservation, you must pick up the permit by 10 a.m on the first day of your planned backcountry stay; otherwise, the permit will be cancelled in its entirety and given to other backpackers. If you know you will not be using your permit, please cancel your reservation as soon as possible.

How to Use the Permit

Your permit is a contract between you and the National Park Service that you agree to treat the backcountry with respect and you will take care of the wilderness.

You will see backcountry regulations on the back of each permit. Read, understand, sign, and obey them. Attach the permit in plain view on the outside of your backpack. When you reach camp, attach the permit to the outside of your tent. The permit indicates the number of people in your party and specifies a campsite for each night you are in the backcountry. You must stick with your planned itinerary so that campsites do not become overcrowded and overused.

Permit Parameters

Individual parties consist of one to seven people. Each party is assigned one campsite.

Each camping area has one to six sites. We recommend you travel in small parties because fewer people per site leaves less impact on RMNP's fragile resources.

Groups consist of 8 to 12 people. They must camp at special group sites. Due to impacts caused by group interaction in and between sites (site spread, social trails etc.), groups of more than seven persons may not camp in neighboring individual sites but must use group sites or split up and camp at least 1 mile apart.

Between June and September, campers may stay in the backcountry for a maximum of seven nights and no more than three consecutive nights in one camp area. Between October and May, campers may stay in the backcountry for a maximum of 14 nights with no more than a total of 21 nights per year.

Setting Out on Your Trip

Always tell someone at home your trip itinerary and when you will return. Allow plenty of time for your trip. Consider the distance you plan to travel, the elevation of the trailhead and your destination, the amount of weight you are carrying, your physical condition, current and forecasted weather, and the hours of daylight remaining.

· Read the trailhead bulletin board.

· Plan to be below tree line during the afternoon when thunderstorms and lightning most often occur.

· Pets, weapons, and vehicles (including mountain bikes) are not allowed in the backcountry.

· Don't forget insect repellent to fend off mosquitoes. Check frequently for ticks.

- Be considerate of others and the resources.
- Set a pace that is comfortable for all members of your party.
- Stay on the trail and hike single file. Resist the temptation to walk off the trail when it is muddy. Mud will flake off your boots much sooner than trampled plants will grow back.
- Never shortcut switchbacks.
- Pick up litter you find along the way.
- Horses and llamas have the right-of-way. Step off the trail on the downhill side and stand quietly until the stock passes.
- Never leave food unattended. Properly store your food.
- Never feed animals.
- When you pause to take a break, sit on rocks or clearings rather than on vegetation.
- Do not disturb any flowers or plants.

Sanitation

There are pit toilets at many backcountry campsites. When a pit toilet is not available, do the following:

- Urinate in rocky places that won't be damaged by animals who dig for the salts and minerals found in urine.
- Dig a hole 6 inches (15 centimeters) deep for solid waste using a small trowel, or pack out waste and paper.
- Be sure that you defecate at least 70 adult steps (200 feet/60 meters) from water or trails.
- Do not bury sanitary napkins or tampons. Dispose of them in an airtight container, and pack them out.
- Wash hands with biodegradable soap. Giardia and other diseases are frequently spread by unsanitary habits.

Please Respect the Fragile Tundra

Alpine-tundra vegetation is hardy. These plants survive extreme cold, strong winds, intense ultraviolet radiation, and very low humidity. Yet, as tough as these plants are, they cannot withstand repeated trampling. It takes 100 years for many alpine-tundra plants to grow an inch.

Where there are no maintained trails and in undeveloped places, you may walk on the alpine tundra, but do not walk in single file. Spread out, so that your footprints are not concentrated on a small area, and rock-hop rather than step on vegetation.

At Camp

When you arrive at your destination, you will see trail signs that show where to find campsites. Pitch your tent in designated areas. Don't pitch your tent on undisturbed vegetation, and never dig or trench around a tent.

There are no grizzly bears in Rocky Mountain National Park, but black bears do live here. Help park rangers keep bears and other animals (including mice, marmots, martens, porcupines, and deer) from becoming a problem by taking precautions with your food and garbage.

- Perhaps the best method to secure your food and scented items is to carry and use a portable food storage container.

- Another method is to hang your food from a tree. The counter balance technique is recommended. Suspend your food at least 10 feet (3 meters) above the ground and 4 horizontal feet (1.5 meters) from the tree trunk. It takes at least 50 feet of rope and two stuff sacks to successfully use this technique. Not all camp areas have trees that are appropriate for hanging items. Inquire at the Backcountry Office.

- Keep a clean camp.

- Seal uneaten food scraps and all garbage in airtight containers or storage bags, and carry all garbage out of the backcountry.

- Refrain from packing greasy, smelly foods into the backcountry.

- Keep all scented items out of your tent including soap, deodorant, and toothpaste. Store them with you food.

  BEWARE: Deer, bighorn sheep, porcupines, and other animals are attracted by sweat and urine. These animals can destroy campsites, clothes, boots, and camping gear in search for salt. Hang your gear and use proper backcountry sanitation.

Preparing Meals at Camp

Cook meals with a portable stove. Do not plan to build a fire. Fires are comforting and aesthetically pleasing, but they cause considerable impact on the backcountry. Wood is better used for habitat for wild creatures than as fuel for campers whose lives do not depend upon forest resources. Campfires have potential to get out of control if not well tended. For these reasons, fires are allowed in only a few designated campsites that have metal fire rings. Never take food in the sleeping area. Separate where you eat from where you sleep.

Drinking Water

Always purify the drinking water you get in the backcountry by using one of the following methods:

- Filter water with a portable purification system that eliminates giardia.

- Boil water for ten minutes.

- Use water-purifying tablets or drops that eliminate giardia.

Wash Water

Carry water at least 70 adult steps (200 feet/60 meters) from a lake or stream to wash yourself or your dishes. Use biodegradable soap. When disposing of wash water, first filter out all food scraps with a small screen. Pack the food scraps into an airtight container to be carried out later. Then toss out the wash water by throwing it over a wide area.

- Never wash directly in a lake or stream.
- Do not scatter food scraps in the water or on the ground.
- Do not throw food into pit toilets.
- Pack out all food scraps, trash, and uneaten food.

Leaving the Backcountry

If you end a trip early, notify a ranger to cancel the permit, so other backpackers may take your place. Please report all unusual wildlife sightings, trail conditions, or incidents to a ranger. Pack out all your garbage and that of others less considerate. If you see any violations of rules and regulations, please report them to a ranger as soon as possible. You can find showers and laundry facilities in Estes Park and in Grand Lake.

Fishing

To fish in Rocky Mountain National Park you must have a Colorado State fishing license. You may purchase licenses at local sporting goods stores. Check at Rocky Mountain National Park visitor centers for fishing regulations. Ask for the Fishing brochure.

Packing with Horses or Llamas

There are special stock campsites and rules for overnight camping with stock. Some trails are closed to stock use. Call (970) 586-1206 or (970) 586-1242 for information about packing with stock. Ask for the "Horse and Pack Animals" brochure.

Check upcoming weather before departing. Remember— conditions can change quickly!

Backcountry Camping Rules and Regulations

A permit is required for all overnight backcountry use and must be displayed on the outside of your pack while you hike to your campsite and also on your tent at the site.

- The permit is valid only for the dates and camp areas listed.
- A displayed dash tag is required for overnight parking.
- Camp must be established on designated tent pads where provided or within 15 feet of the metal arrowhead that marks the designated site.
- Use pit toilets where provided; otherwise, dig a 6-inch-deep "cat hole" at least 200 feet (70 adult steps) from water, trails, and campsites.

General Regulations

In order to protect park resources and minimize impacts, the following are prohibited everywhere in the backcountry:

- Pets, weapons, and vehicles (including bicycles)
- Fires (except at specific sites with metal fire rings)
- Hunting, feeding, approaching, or disturbing wildlife

- Removing or disturbing natural features
- Trenching around tents and camps
- Shortcutting between trail switchbacks
- Littering or leaving trash in sites or pit toilets
- Washing dishes or bathing within 200 feet (70 adult steps) of water.

Special Regulations

DESIGNATED SITES:

- Camp must be established within 15 feet of the metal arrowhead and post that mark the site.

- Use stoves only. Fires prohibited, unless staying in a *wood fire site* with visible metal fire ring (using dead and down wood only).

- Party size is limited to 7 at individual sites and 12 at group sites.

- Due to excessive impact, groups over seven persons must use group sites or split up and camp at least 1 mile apart.

- If the designated site has more than four inches of snow, follow the "Winter Regulations" detailed in a pamphlet available at the backcountry office or online.

Appendix C: Contact Information

NATIONAL PARK SERVICE—ROCKY MOUNTAIN NATIONAL PARK
Estes Park, CO 80517
(970) 586-1206
www.nps.gov/romo
Backcountry information: (970) 586-1242
Recorded information and road and weather
conditions: (970) 586-1333

ESTES PARK CHAMBER OF COMMERCE
(800) 378-3708

ESTES PARK CONVENTION AND VISITORS BUREAU
500 Big Thompson Avenue
P.O. Box 1200
Estes Park, CO 80517
(800) 443-7837
www.estesparkcvb.com

ESTES VALLEY RECREATION AND PARK DISTRICT
690 Big Thompson Avenue
P.O. Box 1379
(970) 586-8191
www.estesvalleyrecreation.com

GRAND LAKE CHAMBER OF COMMERCE
(800) 531-1019

GRAND LAKE CHAMBER OF COMMERCE VISITOR CENTER
P.O. Box 57
Grand Lake, CO 80447
(970) 627-3402
www.grandlakechamber.com

GRAND LAKE METRO RECREATION DISTRICT
P.O. Box 590
Grand Lake, CO 80447
(970) 627-8328

LARIMER COUNTY PARKS AND OPEN LANDS DEPARTMENT
1800 South County Road 31
Loveland, CO 80537
(970) 679-4570
www.larimer.org/parks

ROCKY MOUNTAIN NATURE ASSOCIATION
1895 Fall River Road
Estes Park, CO 80517
(800) 748-7002 or (970) 586-3262
www.rmna.org

U.S. Forest Service: Arapaho and Roosevelt National Forests, Pawnee National Grassland

ROOSEVELT NATIONAL FOREST INFORMATION:
Estes-Poudre Ranger District Office
161 Second Street
P.O. Box 2747
Estes Park, CO 80517
(970) 586-3440

(Continued on next page)

BOULDER RANGER DISTRICT
2140 Yarmouth Avenue
Boulder, CO 80301
(303) 541-2500
www.fs.fed.us/r2/arnf

CANYON LAKES RANGER DISTRICT
2150 Centre Avenue, Building E
Fort Collins, CO 80526
(970) 295-6700
www.fs.fed.us/r2/arnf

PAWNEE NATIONAL GRASSLAND
660 O Street
Greeley, CO 80631
(970) 346-5000
www.fs.fed.us.r2/arnf

SULPHUR RANGER DISTRICT
9 Ten Mile Drive, P.O. Box 10
Granby, CO 80446
(970) 887-4100

Appendix D: Online Map Resources

BRUNTON
www.brunton.com

DELORME
www.delorme.com

EMS
www.ems.com

GARMIN
www.garmin.com

MAGELLAN
www.magellangps.com

MAPQUEST
www.mapquest.com

MAPTECH, INC.
www.maptech.com

MICROSOFT MAPBLAST
www.mapblast.com

NATIONAL GEOGRAPHIC MAPMACHINE
www.nationalgeographic.com/mapmachine

NATIONAL GEOGRAPHIC MAPS
www.nationalgeographic.com/maps

(Continued on next page)

OFFROUTE
www.offroute.com

REI
www.rei.com

SUUNTO
www.suunto.com

TopoZone
www.topozone.com

U.S. FOREST SERVICE
www.fs.fed.us

Maps by phone:
(303) 275-5350
(303) 275-5367 (hearing-impaired)
Maps available at all local agency offices

Maps by mail:
Visitor Map Sales
P.O. Box 25127
Lakewood, CO 80225

U.S. GEOLOGICAL SURVEY
www.usgs.gov

USGS MAP STORE
store.usgs.gov

Appendix E: Web Sites

ACCESS FUND
www.accessfund.org

ACTIVE.COM
www.active.com

AMERICAN HIKING SOCIETY
www.americanhiking.org

AMERICAN TRAILS
www.americantrails.org

AMERICA WALKS
www.americawalks.org

CLIMB THE ROCKIES
www.climbtherockies.com

COLORADO FOURTEENERS INITIATIVE
www.coloradofourteeners.org

COLORADO MOUNTAIN CLUB
www.cmc.org

COLORADO TRAIL FOUNDATION
www.coloradotrail.org

CONTINENTAL DIVIDE TRAIL ALLIANCE
www.cdtrail.org

FOURTEENERS.ORG
www.fourteeners.org

GEOCACHE RESOURCES
www.geocaching.com

(Continued on next page)

Happy Hikers Club
    members.aol.com/happyhikersclub

Hiking and Backpacking
    www.hikingandbackpacking.org/coloradoclubs

Hiking in Colorado
    www.hikingincolorado.org

Letterboxing
    www.letterboxing.org

Mountain Peaks
    www.mountainpeaks.net

Road Runner Club of America
    www.rrca.org

Rocky Mountain Nature Association
    www.rmna.org

Running Network
    www.runningnetwork.com

Run Walk Jog
    www.runwalkjog.com

Sierra Club
    rmc.sierraclub.org

Trails.com
    www.trails.com

Volunteers for Outdoor Colorado
    www.voc.org

Appendix F: **Bibliography**

Dannen, Kent, and Donna Dannen. *Best Easy Day Hikes: Rocky Mountain National Park*. Best Easy Day Hikes Ser. Guilford, CT: Falcon–Globe Pequot, 2002.

Dannen, Kent, and Donna Dannen. *Hiking Rocky Mountain National Park: Including Indian Peaks Wilderness*. 9th ed. Falcon Guides Hiking. Guilford, CT: Falcon–Globe Pequot, 2002.

Donahue, Mike. *The Longs Peak Experience and Trail Guide*. Indiana Camp Supply, 1992.

Dziezynski, James. *Best Summit Hikes in Colorado*. Berkeley: Wilderness Press, 2007.

Fogelberg, Ben, and Steve Grinstead. *Walking into Colorado's Past: 50 Front Range History Hikes*. Englewood, CO: Westcliffe Publishers, 2006.

Foster, Lisa. *Rocky Mountain National Park: The Complete Hiking Guide*. Englewood, CO: Westcliffe Publishers, 2005.

Hailman, Jack, and Elizabeth Hailman. *Hiking Circuits in Rocky Mountain National Park*. Boulder: UP of Colorado, 2003.

Malitz, Jerome. *Rocky Mountain National Park: Dayhiker's Guide*. Rev. ed. Boulder: Johnson, 2005.

Rusk, Dave, and Hal Rusk. *Rocky Mountain Day Hikes: Featuring 24 Hikes in RMNP*. 2nd ed. Estes Park, CO: Barefoot, 1999.

(Continued on next page)

Salcedo, Tracy. *12 Short Hikes: Rocky Mountain National Park Estes Park.* 12 Short Hikes Ser. Guilford, CT: Falcon–Globe Pequot, 1995.

Salcedo, Tracy. *12 Short Hikes: Rocky Mountain National Park Grand Lake.* 12 Short Hikes Ser. Chockstone Press, 1995.

For additional Rocky Mountain National Park books, visit the Rocky Mountain Nature Association's Web site, **www.rmna.org.**

Index

INDEX

part six

About the Author

KIM LIPKER grew up in Colorado loving the outdoors from an early age. She is the author of two other guidebooks for Menasha Ridge Press, *60 Hikes with 60 Miles: Denver and Boulder* and *The Best in Tent Camping: Colorado, 4th Edition* (with Johnny Molloy), along with *The Unofficial Guide to Bed & Breakfasts and Country Inns in the Rockies* (Hungry Minds). She also writes a regular parenting column and other features for *Rocky Mountain Parent* magazine, and she contributes features, ratings, and reviews for Away.com, covering parks, active sports, and outdoor adventures in the Rocky Mountains and Hawaii. Her newest book for Menasha Ridge, *Girls Guide to Hiking and Backpacking,* is scheduled for publication in December 2008.

Considered an expert on the Rocky Mountains by her guidebook peers, Kim has been at the writing thing for a while, having had her first news article published at age 12 and later earning a journalism degree from the University of Missouri–Columbia.

Kim lives in Fort Collins, Colorado, with her husband, Bruce Becker, and her three children, Anna, Alex, and Emma. For more information on her upcoming projects, visit her blog at **trekalong.com/lipker.**

AMERICAN HIKING SOCIETY

Because you hike.

We're with you
every step of the way

American Hiking Society gives voice to the more than
75 million Americans who hike and is the only national
organization that promotes and protects foot trails,
the natural areas that surround them and the hiking
experience. Our work is inspiring and challenging,
and is built on three pillars:

Volunteerism and Stewardship: We organize and
coordinate nationally recognized programs – including
Volunteer Vacations, National Trails Day® and the
National Trails Fund –that help keep our trails open,
safe and enjoyable.

Policy and Advocacy: We work with Congress and
federal agencies to ensure funding for trails, the
preservation of natural areas, and the protection of the
hiking experience.

Outreach and Education: We expand and support
the national constituency of hikers through outreach
and education as well as partnerships with other
recreation and conservation organizations.

**Join us in our efforts. Become an American
Hiking Society member today!**

American
Hiking
Society

1422 Fenwick Lane · Silver Spring, MD 20910 · (301) 565-6704
www.AmericanHiking.org · info@AmericanHiking.org

DEAR CUSTOMERS AND FRIENDS,

SUPPORTING YOUR INTEREST IN OUTDOOR ADVENTURE, travel, and an active lifestyle is central to our operations, from the authors we choose to the locations we detail to the way we design our books. Menasha Ridge Press was incorporated in 1982 by a group of veteran outdoorsmen and professional outfitters. For 25 years now, we've specialized in creating books that benefit the outdoors enthusiast.

Almost immediately, Menasha Ridge Press earned a reputation for revolutionizing outdoors- and travel-guidebook publishing. For such activities as canoeing, kayaking, hiking, backpacking, and mountain biking, we established new standards of quality that transformed the whole genre, resulting in outdoor-recreation guides of great sophistication and solid content. Menasha Ridge continues to be outdoor publishing's greatest innovator.

The folks at Menasha Ridge Press are as at home on a white-water river or mountain trail as they are editing a manuscript. The books we build for you are the best they can be, because we're responding to your needs. Plus, we use and depend on them ourselves.

We look forward to seeing you on the river or the trail. If you'd like to contact us directly, join in at www.trekalong.com or visit us at www.menasharidge.com. We thank you for your interest in our books and the natural world around us all.

SAFE TRAVELS,

Bob Sehlinger

BOB SEHLINGER
PUBLISHER